Physician's Guide to Insulin-Dependent (Type I) Diabetes: Diagnosis and Treatment

7.50

American Diabetes Association, Inc., Alexandria, Virginia 22314

First printing June 1988
Printed in the United States of America
ISBN 0-945448-01-5

Contents

Special Problems

Introduction

The *Physician's Guide to Insulin-Dependent (Type I) Diabetes* is intended to provide primary-care physicians with state-of-the-art practical information on the diagnosis and management of type I diabetes mellitus (IDDM). It is a companion manual to our *Physician's Guide to Non-Insulin-Dependent (Type II) Diabetes.* Together they form the nucleus of the American Diabetes Association's (ADA) Clinical Education Program, an ever-expanding library of professional education materials. Other relevant resources are described in the back of the *Guide.*

Type I diabetes is a chronic disease that often becomes complicated by serious, life-threatening multiorgan dysfunction. In the entire spectrum of diabetes mellitus, prompt diagnosis and treatment of type I is essential to prevent death. Continued close and careful management of the disease is imperative to prevent many of its complications. It is a disease with major psychological ramifications and often imposes considerable life-style impositions throughout life.

ADA is aware that primary-care physicians, who are responsible for the health and well-being of many type I patients, may not be familiar with recently published information or feel confident of managing therapy for these patients. Therefore, the presentation of information about type I diabetes in a clear, concise, and crisp format is essential. The contributors to the *Guide* carefully designed the manuscript to reflect all of the significant aspects of care and management of type I diabetes and to help the practitioner resolve clinical problems and concerns without the burden of excessive background reading.

In almost half a century of leadership in diabetes, ADA's professional education effort has been a major emphasis. We believe that presenting the front-line physician with the most up-to-date information about diabetes will lead to improvements in the health and longevity of individuals with the disease. In this manner, our mission—to promote the search for a preventive and cure for diabetes and to improve the well-being of people with diabetes and their families—moves closer to being fulfilled. We hope this handbook will help and guide you in the treatment of this complex, often complicated disease. In addition, we encourage you to utilize our other clinical education program resources and equally encourage you to contact your local ADA affiliate (see p. 137) to take advantage of ongoing information about diabetes and opportunities to attend our highly regarded professional education meetings.

JOHN A. COLWELL, MD, PhD
President, American Diabetes Association

A Word About This Guide

During the past decade, remarkable progress in the field of diabetes has been rapidly translated into practical advances in patient care. The *Physician's Guide to Insulin-Dependent (Type I) Diabetes* offers state-of-the-art information in a succinct readable form tailored to the needs of the practicing physician. It is not intended as a comprehensive text but as a practical manual on the etiology and management of insulin-dependent diabetes mellitus (type I diabetes mellitus or IDDM), advising clinicians how to provide the best care for patients with type I diabetes and acquainting them with available resources with which to consult or refer.

Type I diabetes is much less common (overall prevalence about 1 in 500) than non-insulin-dependent (type II) diabetes, but its manifestations and effect on the patient are more dramatic. Type I diabetes typically occurs in people less than 30 years old, is the predominant form of diabetes in children and adolescents, may be acutely life threatening in its metabolic derangements at extremes of hypoglycemia and hyperglycemia, and imposes an *absolute dependence on daily injection of insulin for life.* In pregnancy, type I diabetes may jeopardize maternal well-being and fetal outcome. In childhood, it may affect physical and emotional growth. Long-standing disease may be associated with retinopathy, nephropathy, and neuropathy as well as macrovascular complications.

In scope and format, this book emulates *The Physician's Guide to Non-Insulin-Dependent (Type II) Diabetes,* first published in 1984 and revised in 1988. Like its predecessor, it includes the following topics: clinical manifestation at presentation; natural history; management goals; insulin preparations and administration; short- and long-term monitoring of blood glucose; special problems in the adolescent, the elderly, and in pregnancy; and coping skills required of the patient and family. Together, the two *Guides* comprise a current, comprehensive, and clinically useful tool for the treatment of diabetes mellitus.

The guidelines represent the consensus of a panel of authorities expert in the clinical and research aspects of type I diabetes. The work of each contributing editor was extensively discussed by the entire editorial committee at many stages in the development of the manual. A second group of renowned senior consultants further discussed each manuscript and recommended changes. Finally, the views of consultants from other medical specialities that also are involved with managing aspects of type I diabetes were sought.

Therefore, the final product is a highly refined version that constantly emphasizes the practical, highlights recent advances, and suggests future directions. It is intended for the practitioner who may have only a few patients with type I diabetes and who requires resolution of urgent problems and concerns. The discerning reader will note that there are still unanswered questions concerning the diagnosis and treatment of type I diabetes mellitus. We do not, for example, know what causes the disease. We cannot prevent it or its long-term complications. Many of the remaining questions may be resolved in the future. Until then, we expect the *Guide* to become a familiar and trusted friend in your treatment of patients with type I diabetes.

MARK A. SPERLING, MD
Editor-in-Chief

Contributors

Editor-in-Chief

MARK A. SPERLING, MD
Childrens Hospital Medical Center
Cincinnati, Ohio

Contributing Editors

STUART BRINK, MD
New England Diabetes and Endocrinology Center
Chestnut Hill, Massachusetts

DANIEL COX, PhD
University of Virginia Medical Center
Charlottesville, Virginia

RALPH DeFRONZO, MD
Yale University School of Medicine
New Haven, Connecticut

ROBERT N. FRANK, MD
Wayne State University School of Medicine
Detroit, Michigan

STEVEN G. GABBE, MD
Ohio State University
Columbus, Ohio

SAUL M. GENUTH, MD
Case Western Reserve University School of Medicine
Cleveland, Ohio

DAVID GOLDSTEIN, MD
University of Missouri School of Medicine
Columbia, Missouri

DOUGLAS GREENE, MD
University of Michigan Medical Center
Ann Arbor, Michigan

DAVID NATHAN, MD
Massachusetts General Hospital
Boston, Massachusetts

ROBERT RIZZA, MD
Mayo Clinic
Rochester, Minnesota

DAVID SCHADE, MD
University of New Mexico School of Medicine
Albuquerque, New Mexico

MOLLY SOLARES, RN
UCLA School of Medicine
Los Angeles, California

HOPE WARSHAW, MMSc, RD, CDE
Nutrition Consultant
Boston, Massachusetts

Diabetes Consultants

CHARLES M. CLARK, MD
Indiana University School of Medicine
Indianapolis, Indiana

JACQUELINE DUDLEY, RN, CDE
Kilo Diabetes Research Foundation
St. Louis, Missouri

SOLOMON A. KAPLAN, MD
UCLA School of Medicine
Los Angeles, California

ARTHUR KROSNICK, MD
Princeton Diabetes Treatment and Education Center
Princeton, New Jersey

HAROLD E. LEBOVITZ, MD
State University of New York, Health Service Center
Brooklyn, New York

DANIEL PORTE, JR., MD
University of Washington
Seattle, Washington

HAROLD RIFKIN, MD
Albert Einstein College of Medicine
New York, New York

ARLAN L. ROSENBLOOM, MD
University of Florida School of Medicine
Gainesville, Florida

JAY S. SKYLER, MD
University of Miami
Miami, Florida

MADELYN L. WHEELER, MS, RD, CDE
Indiana University Medical Center
Indianapolis, Indiana

Diagnosis and Classification/Pathogenesis

Highlights
Diagnosis and Classification/ Pathogenesis

CLASSIFICATION AND DIAGNOSIS

Diabetes mellitus is classified into three clinically (and possibly pathogenetically) different types:

- **insulin-dependent diabetes (type I or IDDM),**
- **non-insulin-dependent diabetes (type II or NIDDM),** and
- **other types of diabetes,** i.e., diabetes due to or associated with other specific conditions or syndromes.

Diabetes is diagnosed by clinical signs and/or symptoms of

- polyuria,
- polydipsia,
- polyphagia,
- weight loss, and/or
- blurred vision

accompanied by persistent hyperglycemia.

When diabetes is fully evolved, fasting plasma glucose levels exceed 140 mg/dl, and random plasma glucose levels exceed 200 mg/dl.

Incidence of type I diabetes is 15 in 100,000 per year among people under 20 years old, similar in males and females, lower in Blacks than Whites, and markedly less common in Hispanics, Asian Americans, and Native Americans.

At presentation, patients with type I diabetes are usually under 30 years old, lean, and often have experienced significant weight loss, polyuria, and polydipsia before presentation. The oral glucose tolerance test is rarely needed to diagnose type I diabetes.

Delayed diagnosis is a serious, sometimes fatal problem, especially among younger children. Approximately 40% of children under 2 years old present in coma, and of these, approximately 5% die.

Type I diabetes can develop at any age and is sometimes mistaken for type II diabetes among older patients.

PATHOGENESIS

The primary defect in type I diabetes is inadequate insulin secretion by pancreatic beta cells.

Genetic predisposition may play a role in development of some cases of type I diabetes. However, **environmental factors** appear necessary to initiate beta-cell destruction, which is carried out by an autoimmune process not completely understood.

Detectable abnormalities of insulin secretion may be preceded by months to years of beta-cell destruction.

Fasting hyperglycemia occurs when beta-cell mass is reduced by 80 to 90%. Typical symptoms of diabetes, i.e., polyuria, polydipsia, and weight loss, appear once hyperglycemia exceeds the renal threshold of approximately 180 mg/dl glucose.

Sometime after diagnosis and correction of acute metabolic abnormalities, **some individuals experience a "honeymoon phase,"** a temporary period when need for exogenous insulin is diminished or absent.

Within 5 to 10 years after clinical presentation, beta-cell loss is complete; at this point, insulin deficiency is absolute, and circulating islet cell antibodies can no longer be detected.

Classification and Diagnosis

INTRODUCTION

Diabetes mellitus is a chronic disorder that is (1) characterized by hyperglycemia; (2) associated with major abnormalities in carbohydrate, fat, and protein metabolism; and (3) accompanied by a marked propensity to develop relatively specific forms of renal, ocular, neurologic, and premature cardiovascular diseases.

Diabetes encompasses a wide clinical spectrum and is classified into three clinically (and possibly pathogenetically) different types:

- insulin-dependent (type I) diabetes
- non-insulin-dependent (type II) diabetes
- other types of diabetes, i.e., diabetes resulting from or associated with other specific conditions or syndromes.

Although type I accounts for only 10% of all cases of diabetes, its immediate risks and stringent acute treatment requirements demand rapid recognition, diagnosis, and management.

This chapter explores characteristics that differentiate type I from other forms of diabetes, discusses criteria for correct diagnosis, and illustrates various clinical presentations.

CRITERIA FOR DIAGNOSIS

Diabetes is diagnosed by clinical signs and/or symptoms of polyuria, polydipsia, polyphagia, weight loss, and/or blurred vision with persistent hyperglycemia. When diabetes is fully evolved, fasting plasma glucose levels exceed 140 mg/dl, and random plasma glucose levels exceed 200 mg/dl.

If the fasting plasma glucose is below 140 mg/dl, the diagnosis of diabetes may be established by an oral glucose tolerance test (OGTT). An *OGTT is rarely needed to diagnose type I diabetes*. The test now utilizes a 75-gram oral glucose challenge; both the 2-hour plasma glucose value and at least one other value between 0 and 2 hours must exceed 200 mg/dl. Impaired glucose tolerance, as distinguished from diabetes mellitus, refers to abnormal plasma glucose levels that do not meet the criteria for diabetes (Box 1).

RISK OF DEVELOPING TYPE I DIABETES

Type I diabetes accounts for approximately 3% of all new cases of diabetes diagnosed each year in the United States. Although it is much less common in the general population than type II diabetes, type I diabetes is by no means rare among children and young adults. With an estimated annual incidence rate among people under age 20 years of 15 per 100,000 (1 *new* case per 7000 children per yr), type I diabetes is 3- to 4-fold more common than chronic childhood diseases such as cystic fibrosis, peptic ulcer, juvenile rheumatoid arthritis, or leukemia, and it is nearly 10-fold more common than nephrotic syndrome, muscular dystrophy, or lymphoma.

After age 20, the yearly incidence decreases to 5 per 100,000. The incidence is similar in men and women, lower in Blacks than Whites, and markedly less common in Hispanics, Asian Americans, and native Americans. Two to 5% of siblings of individuals with type I diabetes will develop the disorder, and among identical twins, one of whom has type I diabetes, concordance rates are only 50%.

DISTINGUISHING TYPE I DIABETES FROM OTHER FORMS

Type I Diabetes

Type I diabetes can develop at any age, although most cases are generally diagnosed when the patient is less than 30 years old. Because patients with type I diabetes are insulinopenic, insulin therapy is essential to prevent rapid and severe dehydration, catabolism, ketoacidosis, and death. They are usually lean and often have experienced significant weight loss, polyuria, and polydipsia before presentation.

Type II Diabetes

In contrast, patients with type II diabetes generally present after age 30, are not prone to develop ketoacidosis unless

Box 1. Diagnostic Criteria for Diabetes Mellitus, Impaired Glucose Tolerance, and Gestational Diabetes

NONPREGNANT ADULTS

Criteria for Diabetes Mellitus. Diagnosis of diabetes mellitus in nonpregnant adults should be restricted to those who have *one* of the following:

- random plasma glucose level of ≥200 mg/dl *plus* classic signs and symptoms of diabetes mellitus, e.g., polydipsia, polyuria, polyphagia, and weight loss;
- fasting plasma glucose level of ≥140 mg/dl on at least 2 occasions; or
- fasting plasma glucose level <140 mg/dl *plus* sustained elevated plasma glucose levels during at least 2 oral glucose tolerance tests. The 2-h sample and at least one other between 0 and 2 h after 75-g glucose dose should be ≥200 mg/dl. Oral glucose tolerance testing is not necessary if patient has fasting plasma glucose level of ≥140 mg/dl.

Criteria for Impaired Glucose Tolerance. Diagnosis of impaired glucose tolerance in nonpregnant adults should be restricted to those who have *all* of the following:

- fasting plasma glucose of <140 mg/dl;
- 2-h oral glucose tolerance test plasma glucose level between 140 and 200 mg/dl; and
- intervening oral glucose tolerance test plasma glucose level of ≥200 mg/dl.

PREGNANT WOMEN

Criteria for Gestational Diabetes. After an oral glucose load of 100 g, diagnosis of gestational diabetes may be made if 2 plasma glucose values (in mg/dl) equal or exceed

Fasting	1 h	2 h	3 h
105	190	165	145

CHILDREN

Criteria for Diabetes Mellitus. Diagnosis of diabetes mellitus in children should be restricted to those who have *one* of the following:

- random plasma glucose level of ≥200 mg/dl *plus* classic signs and symptoms of diabetes mellitus, e.g., polyuria, polydipsia, ketonuria, and rapid weight loss; or
- fasting plasma glucose level of ≥140 mg/dl on at least 2 occasions *and* sustained elevated plasma glucose levels during at least 2 oral glucose tolerance tests. Both 2-h plasma glucose and at least one other between 0 and 2 h after glucose dose (1.75 g/kg ideal body wt up to 75 g) should be ≥200 mg/dl.

Criteria for Impaired Glucose Tolerance. Diagnosis of impaired glucose tolerance in children should be restricted to those who have *both* of the following:

- fasting plasma glucose concentration <140 mg/dl; and
- 2-h oral glucose tolerance test plasma glucose level of >140 mg/dl.

severely stressed, are generally but not always obese, may be asymptomatic or only mildly symptomatic, and usually have a family history of diabetes. A form of type II diabetes with childhood onset [maturity-onset diabetes of the young (MODY)] is a well-described rare autosomal-dominant disorder.

Patients with type II diabetes are not absolutely dependent on exogenous insulin for survival, although insulin therapy is often employed to lower blood glucose.

Few patients are difficult to categorize as type I or type II. Currently, there is no routinely available test that reliably differentiates between the two types. Generally, if the patient is less than 30 years old, not obese, and has signs and symptoms of diabetes mellitus and an elevated fasting blood glucose, the physician should assume type I diabetes and treat with insulin. The presence of urinary ketones with hyperglycemia in an otherwise unstressed individual strongly supports a diagnosis of type I diabetes, whereas the absence of ketones is of no diagnostic value.

Clinicians should also be aware that some cases presenting as type II diabetes may subsequently be discovered to be type I diabetes (see p. 8 and **Pathogenesis,** p. 11). These patients are usually lean, and their insulin requirements increase as they develop manifestations of complete insulin deficiency.

Some young Black patients present with typical signs and symptoms of type I diabetes but tolerate being off insulin for various periods. They also exhibit evidence of somewhat greater endogenous insulin secretion than most patients with type I diabetes but less than that usually seen in patients with type II diabetes.

The various types of diabetes mellitus and states of impaired glucose tolerance are described in Table 1. Table 2 illustrates specific conditions often associated with the other forms of diabetes and glucose intolerance.

CLINICAL PRESENTATION OF TYPE I DIABETES

The presentation of type I diabetes covers a broad range, from mild nonspecific symptoms to frank coma. In children, correct diagnosis is often delayed because polyuria is incorrectly attributed to urinary tract infection or enuresis; anorexia rather than polyphagia may occur; and fatigue, irritability, weight loss, deterioration of school performance, and enuresis are ascribed to emotional problems. In some cases, failure to thrive may be an overlooked indication of diabetes in a young child.

Fewer patients are presenting with se-

Table 1. Types of Diabetes Mellitus and Other Categories of Glucose Intolerance

CLINICAL CLASSES	DISTINGUISHING CHARACTERISTICS
Diabetes mellitus (DM)	
Insulin-dependent diabetes mellitus (IDDM) Type I	Patients may be of any age, are usually thin, and usually have abrupt onset of signs and symptoms with insulinopenia before age 30 yr. These patients often have strongly positive urine ketone tests in conjunction with hyperglycemia and are dependent on insulin therapy to prevent ketoacidosis and to sustain life.
Non-insulin-dependent diabetes mellitus (NIDDM) Type II (obese or nonobese)	Patients are usually older than 30 yr at diagnosis, obese, and have relatively few classic symptoms. They are not prone to ketoacidosis except during periods of stress. Although not dependent on exogenous insulin for survival, they may require it for adequate control of hyperglycemia.
Other types of diabetes mellitus	Patients with other types of diabetes mellitus have certain associated conditions or syndromes (see Table 3).
Impaired glucose tolerance (IGT) (obese or nonobese)	Patients with impaired glucose tolerance have plasma glucose levels that are higher than normal but not diagnostic for diabetes mellitus.
Other types of impaired glucose tolerance	Patients with other types of impaired glucose tolerance have certain associated conditions or syndromes (see Table 3).
Gestational diabetes mellitus (GDM)	Patients with gestational diabetes mellitus have onset or discovery of glucose intolerance during pregnancy.
STATISTICAL RISK CLASSES*	
Previous abnormality of glucose tolerance (PreAGT)	Patients in this category have normal glucose tolerance and a history of transient diabetes mellitus or impaired glucose tolerance.
Potential abnormality of glucose tolerance (PotAGT)	Patients in this category have never experienced abnormal glucose tolerance but have a greater than normal risk of developing diabetes mellitus or impaired glucose tolerance.

*Used for epidemiologic and research purposes.

Adapted from National Institutes of Health, National Diabetes Data Group: Classification and diagnosis of diabetes mellitus and other categories of glucose intolerance. *Diabetes* 28:1039–57, 1979

Table 2. Other Types of Diabetes Mellitus and Impaired Glucose Tolerance

SECONDARY TO	
Pancreatic disease	**Examples:** pancreatectomy, cystic fibrosis, hemochromatosis, chronic pancreatitis
Endocrinopathies	**Examples:** acromegaly, pheochromocytoma, Cushing's syndrome, primary aldosteronism, glucagonoma
Drugs and chemical agents	**Examples:** certain antihypertensive drugs, thiazide diuretics, glucocorticoids, estrogen-containing preparations, psychoactive agents, catecholamines
ASSOCIATED WITH	
Insulin-receptor abnormalities	**Examples:** acanthosis nigricans
Genetic syndromes	**Examples:** hyperlipidemia, muscular dystrophies, Huntington's chorea
Miscellaneous conditions	**Examples:** malnutrition ("tropical diabetes")

For a more complete list, see National Diabetes Data Group: Classification and diagnosis of diabetes mellitus and other categories of glucose tolerance. *Diabetes* 28:1039–57, 1979

vere metabolic decompensation today than in the past, and more than 70% of cases are diagnosed within 1 month of onset of symptoms. Nevertheless, delayed diagnosis continues to be a serious and sometimes fatal problem, especially among younger children. The frequency of coma as a presenting feature in children less than 2 years old is approximately 40%, compared to less than 10% after 15 years. In children, coma remains an important cause of death; approximately 5% of children presenting in coma die during the acute phase of the disease.

The frequency of various clinical and laboratory characteristics in type I diabetes is shown in Figure 1. In young adults, the presentation is often less acute, although an absolute requirement for insulin becomes evident with time.

CASE PRESENTATIONS

Presentation in Early Childhood

A 19-month-old boy noted by his parents to be extremely fussy was found to be febrile; he had a temperature of 101°F and appeared mildly ill with nasal congestion and a faint pinkish macular rash. A viral respiratory infection was diagnosed, and acetaminophen was prescribed. At home, the fever persisted and occasional vomiting developed.

Two days later, the patient was brought to an emergency room with listlessness and continued vomiting. The child was tachypnic, tachycardic, and dehydrated. Urine was unobtainable, and blood was drawn for a complete blood count (CBC), glucose, and electrolytes. The CBC revealed a white blood cell count (WBC) of 26,000 per cubic millimeter with 70% P, 10% B, 12% L, 8% M, 14.1% hemoglobin, and 48% Hct. Intravenous saline was begun, and because of possible sepsis, a lumbar puncture was done that revealed a clear colorless fluid, slightly elevated protein, and a glucose level of 325 mg/dl.

The blood glucose and electrolyte values were then reported as follows: 650 mg/dl glucose, 129 meq/L Na, 4.5 meq/L K, and 14 meq/L HCO_3. Intravenous insulin was started at 0.1 $U \cdot kg^{-1} \cdot h^{-1}$.* One hour after rehydration with intravenous saline, the child urinated, and rehydration was continued with saline *plus* potassium chloride. Within 6 hours, the infant was clinically improved, the vomiting had stopped, and the pediatric endocrinologist was contacted for ongoing care.

Comment

Onset of type I diabetes is often associated with viral syndromes in this age group. Therefore, the diagnosis of diabetes is often delayed in young children. Infants may develop severe hypertonic dehydration without ketosis, a high-risk situation. When clinical status is out of proportion to the nature of an apparent

*$U \cdot kg^{-1} \cdot h^{-1}$ is often written $U/(kg \cdot h)$ or U/kg/h.

illness, the physician should consider a diagnosis of diabetes mellitus.

Presentation in School-Aged Child

A previously well-adjusted 9-year-old girl was noted to be inattentive in class and easily fatigued. Increased urination and nocturia were overlooked until the family shared a hotel room on a weekend trip, at which time medical attention was sought for a possible bladder infection.

After noting a 3.2-kilogram weight loss, the doctor confirmed the diagnosis of diabetes by documenting glycosuria, ketonuria, and hyperglycemia. Insulin injections twice a day, a balanced meal plan, and self-monitoring of blood glucose (SMBG) were begun.

Comment

Nocturia or recurrence of bed-wetting in a previously toilet-trained child should raise the suspicion of diabetes mellitus. Even with urinary glucose and ketones, a blood glucose test is essential to document hyperglycemia as the cause of glucosuria.

Figure 1. Clinical (*Top*) and Laboratory (*Bottom*) Presentations of Type I Diabetes

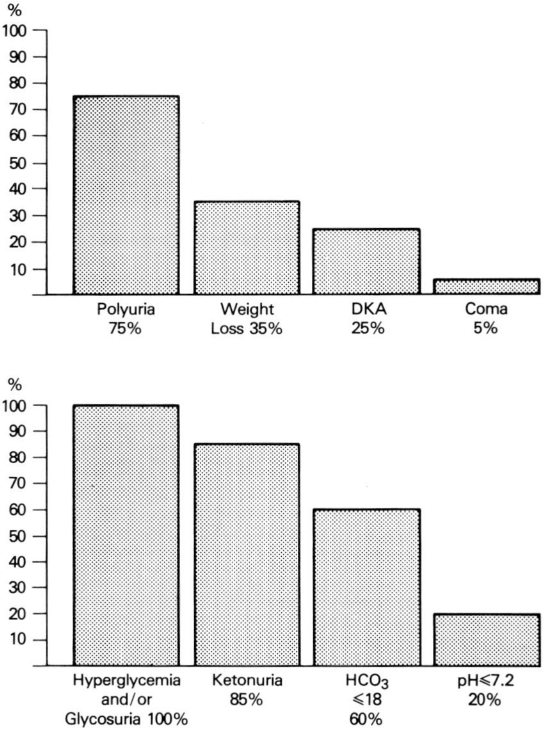

DKA, diabetic ketoacidosis. *Data from* MS Eberhardt, unpublished observations

Presentation in Adolescence

A 15-year-old girl was delighted to be losing weight, although she felt abnormally tired and thirsty, had been urinating frequently during the day for 2 weeks, and had developed a white pruritic vaginal discharge, which she discussed with her mother and a friend.

A visit to the doctor disclosed that she had lost 6.4 kilograms. *Candida albicans* was cultured, and glycosuria and small ketonuria were noted. Blood glucose was elevated, confirming the diagnosis, but serum electrolytes were normal. Diabetes education was started, and insulin injections prebreakfast and at bedtime were begun.

Comment

Unexplained weight loss, increased urination, or a vaginal infection in an adolescent should raise the possibility of diabetes.

Presentation in Young Adulthood

A 23-year-old nonobese man noted fatigue, blurred vision, polyuria, and polydipsia without polyphagia for 1 week. His father, a physician, diagnosed diabetes on the basis of a random blood glucose level of 325 mg/dl.

Despite the absence of obesity and a recent 2.2-kilogram weight loss, an 800-calorie diet was prescribed. Two weeks later, in the face of continued polyuria, polydipsia, malaise, and an additional 6.8-kilogram weight loss, an oral sulfonylurea was prescribed and was increased to a maximal dosage over the succeeding month.

An additional month of treatment with maximal dosages of a second-generation sulfonylurea was accompanied by a further loss of 4.5 kilograms and the development of malaise and mild nausea without vomiting. The patient was eventually referred to the hospital for admission.

Somnolence and dry mucus membranes were noted. Pulse was 90 beats per minute, and blood pressure was 110/65 mmHg sitting and 100/50 mmHg standing. Skin turgor was decreased. Mild diffuse abdominal tenderness without rebound and tender hepatomegaly were present. Urinalysis was 4+ for glucose, large for ketones, and negative for protein. The following results were found: 520 mg/dl blood glucose, 145 meq/L Na, 5.0 meq/L K, 110 meq/L Cl, and 20 meq/L HCO_3. Hematocrit was 53%, and WBC count was 12,500 per cubic millimeter without a left shift. Arterial pH was 7.30. Plasma ketones were present.

A diagnosis of type I diabetes with ketosis was made, and the patient was begun on an insulin infusion that rapidly reversed signs and symptoms of hyperglycemia and laboratory abnormalities. He was discharged on a regimen of mixed NPH and regular insulin twice daily and entered a diabetes education program. He regained most of his lost weight and returned to work.

Comment

Physicians often mistake type I for type II diabetes in older patients. Type I diabetes can occur at any age and should be considered in nonobese people with signs and symptoms of diabetes and an elevated fasting blood glucose, especially with weight loss and ketonuria. Such patients may become very dehydrated despite the absence of severe acidosis. *Dietary restriction and sulfonylureas are ineffective in controlling the metabolic abnormalities of type I diabetes and should not be used.*

Presentation in a Patient Over 40 Years Old

A 59-year-old woman with a strongly positive family history of type II diabetes presented with polydipsia and polyuria. She was not overweight. For 11 years she was successfully treated with diet and chlorpropamide, during which time her weight remained stable and she was free of symptoms of hyperglycemia.

At age 70, she again developed polydipsia and polyuria and lost 4.5 kilograms. Therapy was changed to 24 units of NPH insulin subcutaneously each morning, and she regained weight to 52 kilograms and remained free of symptoms.

At age 82, the polydipsia and polyuria recurred, and a 4.5-kilogram weight loss was noted. Evening NPH and morning and evening regular insulin were added to her regiman, with little effect. On four occasions over the next 6 months, she was admitted to the hospital with diabetic ketoacidosis, for which no precipitating causes or stresses could be identified.

She was finally begun on a program of SMBG four times daily with mixed intermediate- and short-acting insulins before breakfast, short-acting insulin before dinner, and intermediate-acting insulin at bedtime. After treatment, fasting glucose was 142 mg/dl, and endogenous insulin secretion assessed by C-peptide was less than 0.1 ng/ml (normal 0.8–4.0 ng/ml).

Comment

The patient probably had very slowly evolving type I diabetes. The presence of both type I and type II diabetes in the same family is not unusual.

CONCLUSION

Patients with type I diabetes are dependent on insulin for life—to live and for as long as they live. Any lean individual less than 30 years old with typical signs and symptoms of hyperglycemia should be assumed to have type I diabetes. A high index of suspicion is needed to diagnose diabetes in very young children or elderly patients.

Pathogenesis

INTRODUCTION

The primary defect in insulin-dependent (type I) diabetes mellitus is inadequate insulin secretion by pancreatic beta cells, which results in hyperglycemia, polyuria, polydipsia, and weight loss. Clinical onset may be preceded by an extensive asymptomatic period during which beta cells are continuously destroyed. Loss of remaining beta cells progresses even after clinical presentation and ultimately becomes complete. The evolving process of beta-cell destruction, with progressive insulin loss, gives rise to a broadly predictable pattern of glucose homeostasis both before and for some time after diagnosis of diabetes.

ROLE OF INSULIN

As the chief modulator of nutrient disposition, storage, and release, plasma insulin concentration influences various anabolic and catabolic processes. The rise in plasma insulin after a meal stimulates storage of glucose as glycogen in liver and muscle; it enhances fat deposition in adipose tissue, inhibits protein degradation, and accelerates the processes of amino acid transport into cells and protein synthesis. The fall in insulin level during normal overnight fasting facilitates the release of stored glucose from liver, protein from muscle, and fat from adipose tissue.

In normal individuals, there is fluctuation between the high-insulin (anabolic) phase during feeding and the low-insulin (catabolic) phase during fasting. In contrast, patients with type I diabetes are in a state of permanent, severe, fasting catabolism. Their eventual absolute lack of insulin causes inability to store exogenous nutrients and uncontrolled release of stored nutrients from liver, muscle, and adipose tissue (Table 3).

Normal Glucose Homeostasis

During fasting, the primary determinant of blood glucose concentration is the rate of basal hepatic glucose production. When food is not being ingested, e.g., after the evening meal and throughout the sleeping hours, the adult liver adds glucose to the circulation at a rate (~2 $mg \cdot kg^{-1} \cdot min^{-1}$*) that precisely matches the rate of peripheral, largely cerebral, glucose utilization. By this means, the fasting plasma glucose concentration is maintained constant at an average level of 80 to 90 mg/dl. The normal rate of hepatic glucose production is of critical importance because the cerebral tissues are dependent on glucose as a metabolic fuel.

The rise in blood glucose after nutrient ingestion stimulates release of insulin. As glucose enters the circulation from the gastrointestinal tract, two insulin-regulated processes act to restrain the rise in blood glucose concentration: suppression of hepatic glucose output and stimulation of glucose uptake via muscle and liver. Secreted insulin is carried via the portal circulation to the liver where about half of it binds to receptors on the hepatocyte, signaling suppression of hepatic glucose production. The remaining half passes to the peripheral circulation where it stimulates glucose uptake, primarily by muscle tissue.

NATURAL HISTORY OF BETA-CELL DEFECT

Current thought on the evolution of frank diabetes includes (Figure 2)

- genetic predisposition;
- precipitating events of uncertain type;
- progressive autoimmune destruction of pancreatic beta cells, eventually resulting in
  - loss of first-phase insulin response to intravenous glucose, followed by
  - progressive impairment in the total insulin response, leading to
  - clinically detectable hyperglycemia.

Genetic Predisposition

The histocompatibility leukocyte antigen (HLA) complex, located on chro-

*$mg \cdot kg^{-1} \cdot min^{-1}$ is often written $mg/(kg \cdot min)$ or mg/kg/min.

Table 3. Physiologic Effects of High- Versus Low-Insulin States

	HIGH-INSULIN (FED) STATE	LOW-INSULIN (FASTED) STATE
Liver	Glucose uptake Glycogen synthesis Lipogenesis Absent ketogenesis Absent gluconeogenesis	Glucose production Glycogenolysis Absent lipogenesis Ketogenesis Gluconeogenesis
Muscle	Glucose uptake Glucose oxidation Glycogen synthesis Protein synthesis	Absent glucose uptake Fatty acid oxidation Ketone oxidation Glycogenolysis Proteolysis and amino acid release
Adipose tissue	Glucose uptake Lipid synthesis Triglyceride uptake	Absent glucose uptake Lipolysis and fatty acid release Absent triglyceride uptake

mosome 6, consists of a cluster of genes that code for transplantation antigens and regulation of the immune response. Inheritance of certain HLA types, principally the DR3 and DR4 loci, confers a tendency to develop type I diabetes.

Either the DR3 or DR4 locus, or both, is present in approximately 95% of patients with type I diabetes. Inheritance of one of these antigens increases the risk of developing type I 3- to 5-fold. When both are present, risk increases 10- to 20-fold over that of the general population.

Inheritance studies of families with a diabetic member clearly document the importance of the HLA region in determining who will develop diabetes. If one sibling has type I diabetes, the risk that another will develop the disease is directly proportional to the number of HLA haplotypes they share. If two haplotypes are shared, the risk is 1 in 5; if one haplotype is shared, the risk is 1 in 20; if no haplotypes are shared, the risk drops to 1 in 100. Overall, only about 5% of siblings of an index case will develop type I diabetes mellitus.

Genetic factors alone are inadequate to cause type I diabetes; i.e., it is the tendency and not the disease itself that is inherited. The fact that identical twins are concordant for type I diabetes only 50% of the time suggests that some environmental factor(s) is needed to initiate the disease process. These factors and their mode of action remain unknown. Several causative agents including viruses and drugs have been proposed, but none has gained widespread acceptance.

Progressive Autoimmune Beta-Cell Destruction

In most patients, strong evidence implicates an autoimmune process in beta-cell destruction. This evidence includes

- greater-than-chance association of type I with some autoimmune diseases,
- association of diabetes genes and HLA region,
- presence at diagnosis of anti-islet cell and anti-insulin antibodies,
- presence at diagnosis of inflammatory cells around islets, and
- activation of T-lymphocytes, including presence of Ia-positive T-lymphocytes.

Because insulin secretory reserves are considerable, individuals who develop type I diabetes go through a variable interval of months to years with no detectable abnormalities in insulin secretion or glucose metabolism despite ongoing destruction of beta-cell mass.

Earliest Abnormalities in Insulin Response

The earliest detectable abnormality in insulin secretion is a progressive reduction of the immediate (first-phase) plasma insulin response during intra-

Figure 2. Proposed Scheme of Natural History of Beta-Cell Defect

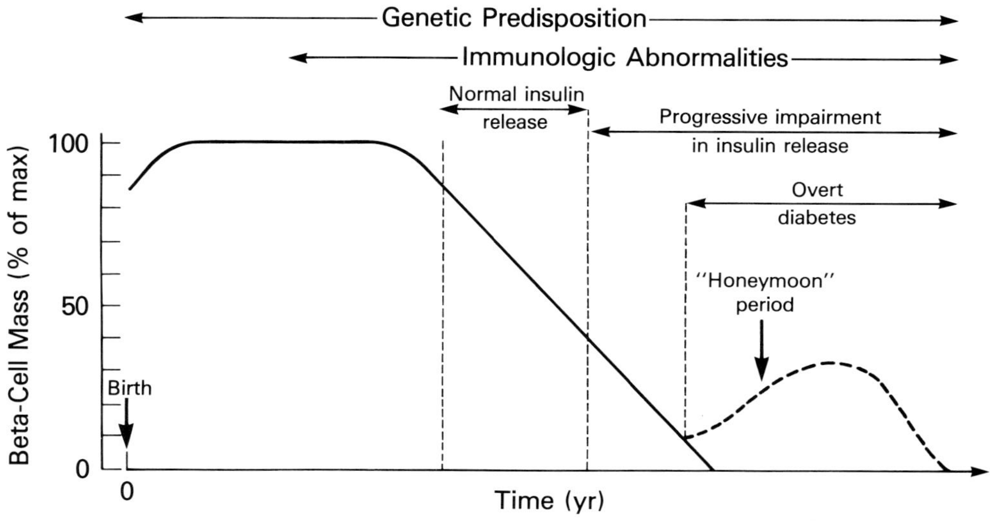

Timing of trigger in relation to immunologic abnormalities is unknown. Note that overt diabetes is not apparent until insulin secretory reserves are <10–20% of normal.

venous glucose tolerance testing. This impairment alone has little deleterious effect on overall glucose homeostasis: fasting plasma glucose concentration is normal, and the response to an oral glucose challenge is virtually unimpaired. At this stage of the evolution of the disease, most affected individuals have circulating antibodies to islet cells or to their own insulin, a finding extremely rare in the general population. Although these antibodies appear to be markers for ongoing beta-cell damage, assays for them are not sufficiently standardized to be clinically useful at present.

Overt glucose intolerance emerges when insulin secretory reserves are reduced to less than 20% of normal. At this point, all phases of the insulin secretory response are reduced so that hepatic glucose production becomes excessive, glucose uptake by peripheral tissues is lowered, and the oral glucose tolerance test (OGTT) becomes abnormal.

Some patients who appear to have non-insulin-dependent (type II) diabetes, with its less severe disturbance in carbohydrate metabolism and its freedom from ketosis under basal conditions, may in fact be in an early stage of evolving type I diabetes.

Clinical Onset

When ongoing destruction has reduced beta-cell mass by 80 to 90%, fasting hyperglycemia, which results chiefly from unrestrained hepatic glucose production, and marked glucose intolerance ensue.

Once hyperglycemia exceeds the renal threshold of approximately 180 mg/dl glucose, glucosuria and osmotic diuresis result in the typical symptoms of polyuria, compensatory polydipsia, and weight loss. If untreated, excessive fluid and electrolyte losses occur. With evolving insulin deficiency and/or pathophysiologic stress, plasma concentrations of glucagon, growth hormone, epinephrine, and cortisol increase. These hormones antagonize insulin's effect, further promoting gluconeogenesis, glycogenolysis, lipolysis, and ketogenesis. Unrestrained ketogenesis and acid-base disturbances result in frank diabetic ketoacidosis.

At initial presentation with symptomatic hyperglycemia or ketoacidosis, circulating insulin levels are low or undetectable, and there is no significant beta-cell response to any of the usual insulin secretagogues. Insulin requirements are relatively large, partly owing to lack of insulin secretion, and partly to a modest degree of insulin resistance.

HONEYMOON PHASE

Somewhat later, once metabolic derangements are corrected, significant residual insulin secretion can often be demonstrated, indicating that some beta-cell reserve remains. As spontaneous insulin secretion becomes evident, exogenous insulin requirements may decrease dramatically, and some diabetic individuals may even temporarily cease to require insulin (honeymoon period). It is unusual for the honeymoon period to last for more than several months to 1 year, and the need for exogenous insulin replacement becomes inevitable.

Because of the evidence for an autoimmune process in the gradual destruction of beta cells and the evidence for residual insulin secretory reserves at clinical presentation, several immune therapies have been attempted to preserve remaining beta cells. Although some of the therapies have temporarily maintained endogenous insulin secretion to the point of permitting discontinuation of exogenous insulin, none has caused permanent remission.

Additionally, the side effects of these therapies have been considerable and fraught with the dangers of overall immune suppression. Hence, all therapies, including cyclosporin, have a large risk-to-benefit ratio, remain experimental, and cannot be routinely recommended for newly diagnosed patients.

Within 5 to 10 years after clinical presentation, beta-cell loss is complete. At this point, insulin deficiency is absolute and circulating islet cell antibodies can no longer be detected.

CONCLUSION

Individuals who are genetically or otherwise predisposed to develop type I diabetes eventually demonstrate near-total failure of insulin secretion as the result of an immunologically mediated progressive destruction of beta-cell mass. The emergence of insulinopenia is associated with several intracellular abnormalities in both liver and muscle tissue, leading to excessive hepatic glucose production, decreased muscle glucose uptake, frank glucose intolerance and, if untreated, ketoacidosis. *Because insulin deficiency is primary, patients are dependent on exogenous insulin for life.*

BIBLIOGRAPHY

Barrett E, DeFronzo RA: Diabetic ketoacidosis. *Hosp Pract* 19:89–104, 1984

Eisenbarth GS: Type I diabetes mellitus: a chronic autoimmune disorder. *N Engl J Med* 314:1360–68, 1986

Eisenbarth GS, Connelly J, Soeldner JS: The "natural" history of type I diabetes. *Diabetes Metab Rev* 3:873–92, 1987

Gepts W, In't Veld PA: Islet morphologic changes. *Diabetes Metab Rev* 3:859–72, 1987

Lernmark Å: Molecular biology of type I (insulin-dependent) diabetes mellitus. *Diabetologia* 28:195–203, 1985

Nerup J, Mandrup-Poulsen T, Molvig J: The HLA-IDDM association: implications for etiology and pathogenesis of IDDM. *Diabetes Metab Rev* 3: 779–802, 1987

Riley WJ, Winter WE, Maclaren NK: Identification of insulin-dependent diabetes mellitus before onset of clinical symptoms. *J Pediatr* 112:314–16, 1988

Routine Management: Objectives

Highlights
Routine Management: Objectives

PHILOSOPHY AND GOALS

Three factors strongly influence treatment:

- **the physician's treatment philosophy,** including beliefs regarding glycemic control and complications
- **the patient's self-care attitudes and abilities**
- **physician-patient congruence of goals.**

Evidence relating glycemic control to later complications should be carefully considered by physicians. Evidence from many sources, including animal models, kidney transplants, and retrospective and prospective studies of glycemic control in humans, is summarized on pages 15–16.

The physician and patient must set treatment goals together with the health-care team and family.

Educational goals are defined on page 17. They cover the broad areas of

- pathophysiology;
- skills relating to insulin, monitoring, food, and exercise; and
- enlisting the help of others to deal with hypoglycemia and impending ketoacidosis.

Clinical goals are presented on page 17. At diagnosis, they include

- metabolic stabilization,
- restoration of desirable body weight, and
- elimination of hyperglycemic symptoms.

Ongoing clinical goals relate to

- maintenance of normal physical and psychosocial functioning and
- minimizing the adverse impact of diabetes on the patient's life.

Treatment goals will differ from patient to patient. Descriptions of minimal, average, and intensive control of diabetes are presented in Box 2, page 18.

EDUCATION

Appropriate diabetes education teaches the patient how to incorporate diabetes management into daily life and to minimize dependence on the physician.

Before teaching can begin, crucial information about the patient must be obtained. Areas that should be assessed at the first interview are covered on page 21. The educator should also allay anxiety, identify areas of misinformation, and elicit attitudes toward diabetes.

Effective teaching requires adequate time. However, short, well-reinforced lessons plus close phone contact to answer "real-life" questions are preferable to lengthy classroom sessions. **Oral instructions should be supported with concise written explanations.**

Survival skills must be learned with 100% accuracy, preferably by both patient and family, because the patient's life depends on those skills. Survival skills are listed in Box 4, page 22.

In-depth education should begin within 3 to 4 weeks of diagnosis. Topics are covered in detail on pages 25–27. Learning must be evaluated over both the short and long term.

Philosophy and Goals

INTRODUCTION

Insulin-dependent (type I) diabetes mellitus is a prime example of a disease in which the goals and attitudes of the physician, coupled with those of the patient, are paramount in determining management and outcome. Three factors that strongly influence treatment are

- the physician's treatment philosophy, including beliefs regarding glycemic control and complications;
- the patient's self-care attitudes and abilities; and
- physician-patient congruence of goals.

PHILOSOPHY OF TREATMENT

For the physician, the primary aim of treatment must be to restore patients to a state of day-to-day clinical well-being and keep them there, free from the threat of metabolic disequilibrium and its serious consequences. The secondary aim of treatment is to prevent, delay, or arrest the vascular complications facing most patients who have had the disease for 10 to 20 years. The first aim is clearly achievable at reasonable degrees of cost, inconvenience, and risk; the second is much more problematic.

Evidence relating hyperglycemia and/or other metabolic consequences of insulin deficiency to the development of vascular complications is not totally conclusive. No particular level of metabolic control has been demonstrated to prevent or arrest these complications in patients with type I diabetes. Furthermore, intensified treatment techniques seldom truly normalize the metabolic environment, but they increase the risk of hypoglycemia and require extraordinary effort and commitment from the patient and health-care team.

However, evidence for a link between glycemic control and complications is persuasive enough to warrant the multimillion-dollar Diabetes Control and Complications Trial (DCCT), sponsored by the National Institutes of Health. The DCCT is a long-term, prospective, randomized, controlled, multicenter trial studying the course of approximately 1400 patients with type I diabetes. These patients are treated with intensive or conventional insulin regimens. The DCCT is designed to answer two questions: whether intensive glycemic control can prevent microvascular disease from developing at all and whether it can arrest or reverse *early* microvascular complications already present (with retinopathy as the primary endpoint). When it is completed in the early 1990s, the DCCT should provide, for the first time, a solid foundation for treatment decisions.

Until then, the level of metabolic control sought must take into consideration both the patient's capabilities and the physician's beliefs regarding the role of glycemic control in preventing complications. Available evidence (summarized below) should be carefully considered by each physician and health-care team member and discussed in appropriate terms with patients and their families.

GLYCEMIC CONTROL AND COMPLICATIONS: A SUMMARY OF EVIDENCE

Animal Studies

Strong experimental support for an association between metabolic abnormalities and vascular complications is found in animal studies. Animals that are rendered insulin deficient and hyperglycemic develop pathologic changes resembling early human retinopathy and nephropathy and functional changes resembling human neuropathy. These changes can be prevented or ameliorated and, in some instances, even reversed by intensive insulin treatment, by cure of diabetes through pancreas transplantation in inbred strains, or by transplant of the affected organ into a nondiabetic animal. However, neither proliferative retinopathy severe enough to impair vision nor renal insufficiency of a degree that would shorten life has ever developed in the diabetic models, perhaps because of inadequate time or variation in species susceptibility. Therefore, the most critical animal test of the glucose hypothesis has not been possible.

Human Diabetes Resulting From Islet Destruction

Microvascular disease also develops in some patients with diabetes resulting from removal or destruction of the islets because of pancreatectomy, chronic pancreatitis, or toxicity (e.g., from the rodenticide Vacor). These observations further support the thesis that loss of insulin secretion or some consequent metabolic derangement is responsible for microvascular abnormalities in patients with idiopathic type I diabetes.

Kidney Transplantation Observations

Normal kidneys transplanted into recipients with type I diabetes begin to show pathologic changes resembling diabetic nephropathy after several years, again pointing to a causative role for the diabetic metabolic milieu.

Retrospective Human Studies

Certain retrospective studies in type I patients suggest that the higher the previous levels of glycemia, the greater the incidence of microvascular disease found on survey. Studies have not been completely conclusive, which may be attributable to imperfect methods of achieving and quantitating metabolic control and to potential bias induced by patient self-selection in the type of treatment.

Prospective Human Studies

Prospective human studies have been inconclusive. Up to 3 years of intensive insulin treatment, with resultant lower blood glucose levels, has not shown a clear beneficial effect on the progression of already established retinopathy or clinically significant nephropathy. In fact, temporary worsening of retinopathy in the first 6 to 12 months of treatment has been reported.

These negative results need not preclude a beneficial effect of intensive treatment extended over a longer time or begun before complications are established. Recent reports that such treatment may halt progression of early microalbuminuria suggest its potential value, again emphasizing the importance of the DCCT study.

Other Factors

Some patients with type I diabetes never develop clinically significant retinopathy, and many never develop renal insufficiency, apparently regardless of their previous levels of metabolic control. This and several other observations imply that additional factors, perhaps *genetic,* may predispose to or protect against the development of particular complications.

GOALS OF TREATMENT

The physician and patient, with the health-care team and family, must set treatment goals *together.* This deceptively simple point often leads to failure if overlooked. The physician bent on tight control in every case will only be frustrated by a patient who does not understand the need for, or is unwilling to accept, the goal. Conversely, the patient who wants blood glucose normal all the time and is truly willing to work for it will be frustrated by a physician who lacks the time, the facilities, the conviction, or the training to help achieve this goal.

In addition to a clear agreement on goals, a good physician-patient treatment match requires open communication and appropriate patient education. At the tightest end of the treatment spectrum, the patient must have a sophisticated understanding of physiology to maintain normal glycemia when, for example, exercising strenuously. In contrast, at the looser end, knowledge may be more rudimentary, but patients must at least know that to avoid diabetic ketoacidosis (DKA), they may have to take extra insulin on sick days when appetite is poor and common sense might dictate the reverse. Treatment must always be individualized with regard to specific goals; sometimes more can be gained by striving for less.

The physician and team members should avoid seeming autocratic, moralistic, or judgmental. They should try to hide their disappointment when goals are not met easily or quickly and should empathize with the patient's difficulty in paying daily attention to the unceasing demands of diabetes. It is important to encourage the best goals achievable without demanding the impossible.

The following educational and clinical goals are appropriate for all patients with type I diabetes.

EDUCATIONAL GOALS

The patient and family should understand the basic pathophysiology of type I diabetes. The patient and family should learn to

- administer insulin,
- monitor blood and urine glucose,
- measure urine ketones,
- select foods and estimate quantities,
- prevent and treat hypoglycemia, and
- adjust insulin, food intake, or both for changes in usual exercise and eating patterns.

School nurses, roommates, employers, and fellow employees should learn to recognize the symptoms of hypoglycemia and impending ketoacidosis and to respond appropriately. The patient should understand how to decrease morbidity from established retinopathy, neuropathy, peripheral vascular disease, hypertension, and nephropathy (see **Education** for details).

CLINICAL GOALS

Initial Goals

For the new-onset, acutely decompensated patient or the previously diagnosed patient in blatantly poor control, goals should include

- elimination of ketosis;
- a return to desirable body weight range by
    - reversing water and extracellular electrolyte losses,
    - replenishing lean body mass (protein and intracellular electrolytes), and
    - returning fat stores to 10 to 20% of total weight; and
- elimination of obvious consequences of hyperglycemia, e.g., gross polyuria and polydipsia, vaginitis or balanitis, recurrent infections, and visual blurring.

Further Goals

Once the above has been achieved, further goals should include the following.

- Preventing urinary frequency and thirst from disturbing sleep, school, work, social, or recreational activities.
- Preventing spontaneous and aborting illness-induced ketonuria.
- Maintaining weight within desirable range.
- Stimulating catch-up growth and sexual maturation in poorly controlled children.
- Maintaining normal growth rate in children and adolescents.
- Maintaining maximum exercise tolerance and stamina.
- Maintaining sense of well-being and self-worth, normal initiative, normal desire for socialization, and freedom from morbid thoughts.
- Minimizing self-treatable hypoglycemia and avoiding hypoglycemic seizures, accidents (e.g., while driving), and coma.
- Avoiding hospitalization.
- For women, achieving normal fertility and pregnancy outcome.
- Sustaining normal family and marital relationships and sex life.
- Preventing diabetes-dictated or diabetes-oriented life-style (i.e., diabetes controlling the patient rather than vice versa).

LEVELS OF TREATMENT

In addition to the educational and clinical goals discussed above, patients and physicians should work toward goals of diabetes control. The goals may be characterized in terms of three *levels of treatment*—minimal, average, and intensive—each having a typical biochemical and clinical profile (Box 2).

Assessors of Control

Diabetes control is generally assessed at home via self-monitoring of blood glucose (SMBG) and/or urine glucose, and in the office it is assessed by results of glycohemoglobin tests. Although office-monitored results ideally should agree with SMBG and urine tests, in practice, correlation with frequently determined SMBG is quite good, whereas correlation with urine tests is poor. Glycosyl-

Box 2. Levels of Treatment: Biochemical and Clinical Characteristics

Minimal
- HbA_{1c} 11.0–13.0% and GHb 13.0–15.0%
- Many SMBG values of ≥300 mg/dl
- Almost constantly positive urine glucose tests
- Intermittent spontaneous ketonuria

Average
- HbA_{1c} 8.0–9.0% and GHb 10.0–11.0%
- Premeal SMBG 160–200 mg/dl
- Intermittent positive urine glucose
- Rare ketonuria

Intensive
- HbA_{1c} 6.0–7.0% and GHb 7.0–9.0%
- Premeal SMBG 70–120 mg/dl; postmeal SMBG <180 mg/dl
- Essentially no positive urine glucose or ketones

ated hemoglobin values are expressed in two ways corresponding to the most commonly available types of assays: hemoglobin A_{1c} (HbA_{1c}) and either HbA_1 or total glycosylated hemoglobin (GHb) (see **Monitoring,** p. 44). In absolute terms, HbA_1 or GHb values are generally 1.0 to 2.0% greater than HbA_{1c} values.

Generally, a 1% change in glycosylated hemoglobin levels corresponds to a change in mean blood glucose of 35 mg/dl. In nondiabetic individuals, glycosylated hemoglobin ranges are 4.0 to 6.0% HbA_{1c} and 5.0 to 8.0% GHb. These correspond to mean blood glucose levels of about 90 mg/dl.

When these data were compiled, patients with type I diabetes in the United States averaged 8.0 to 9.0% HbA_{1c} and 10.0 to 11.0% GHb. These correspond to mean blood glucose levels of about 200 mg/dl. Adolescents average a 1% increase and blood glucose of 40 mg/dl higher than adults. Ninety-five percent of type I patients have glycosylated hemoglobin values of 5.0 to 13.0% HbA_{1c} and 6.0 to 15.0% GHb. Levels as high as 20 to 25% are seen in newly diagnosed and other poorly controlled patients.

Results of Minimal Treatment

With a minimal level of treatment, glycosylated hemoglobin can be expected to be maintained at 11.0 to 13.0% HbA_{1c} and 13.0 to 15.0% GHb. These patients can be expected to have many SMBG values of 300 mg/dl and higher, almost constantly positive urine glucose tests, and intermittent spontaneous ketonuria. They will also have symptoms of polyuria and polydipsia (that may not be noticed or admitted to) and a growth pattern that is probably slower than would otherwise be genetically determined. On the other hand, at this level of control, DKA can usually be avoided, and patients can generally function in some fashion at home, work, or school.

A minimal level of treatment may be the best that can be achieved in some adolescents and in a few nonadherent adults. However, it should never be accepted as a goal unless health-care team efforts to improve alienate the patient, make routine follow-up care impossible, and make emergency care the rule. (Note that because blood glucose levels tend to rise with age in nondiabetic subjects, the elderly patient with 10% HbA_{1c} and 12% GHb may be considered to be closer to an average than a minimal level of treatment.)

Results of Average Treatment

With an average level of treatment, glycosylated hemoglobin is maintained at 8.0 to 10.0% HbA_{1c} and 10.0 to 12.0% GHb. These patients can be expected to have average premeal blood glucose levels of 160 to 200 mg/dl, intermittently positive urine glucose, and only rare ketonuria. They will experience little or no polyuria or polydipsia, maintain body weight, exhibit normal-range growth rates, and usually appear to function normally in daily living. They will probably average one self-treated hypoglycemic reaction a week, and 10% will suffer one severe reaction a year. Achieving at least this result ensures the patient of a state of acceptable clinical well-being and offers the satisfaction of knowing that this individual is doing better than half of all patients with type I diabetes.

Results of Intensive Treatment

At an intensive level of treatment, glycosylated hemoglobin levels are usually maintained at 6.0 to 7.0% HbA_{1c} and 7.0 to 9.0% GHb, i.e., just above values for nondiabetic people. The patients will have premeal blood glucose levels of 70 to 120 mg/dl, postmeal blood glucose values of less than 180 mg/dl, and essentially no positive urine glucose or ketones. They are entirely asymptomatic from hyperglycemia and may perceive improvement in their general sense of well-being, energy, exercise capacity, disease-related anxiety and affect, compared with maintenance at considerably higher glycosylated hemoglobin levels. However, they may experience increased mild self-treated hypoglycemic reactions and severe hypoglycemic episodes. They may also find the required frequent monitoring, insulin administration methods, and constant dietary adherence to be excessively burdensome.

APPROPRIATE TREATMENT GOALS FOR ALL PATIENTS

The following goals are appropriate for patients with type I diabetes.

- In all patients, seek the fullest possible educational and clinical goals.
- In all pregnant women and women attempting to conceive, seek stringent biochemical goals of intensive treatment (5.5–6.5% HbA_{1c} and 5.5–7.0% GHb, blood glucose 60–110 mg/dl) by methods detailed below (see **Pregnancy,** p. 80).
- In other type I patients who are well-informed about the risks and potential benefits of intensive therapy, highly motivated, and suitably educable, seek an intensive level of treatment (6.0–7.0% HbA_{1c} and 7.0–9.0% GHb). However, if the patients do not sense or respond to hypoglycemia, goals should be set higher.
- In all patients on conventional two-injection insulin regimens, seek at least the average level of treatment (8.0–9.0% HbA_{1c} and 10.0–11.0% GHb).
- Generally, the greater the physician's and patient's belief in preventing vascular complications by tight control, the lower the mutually set targets should be.

CONCLUSION

For patients with type I diabetes, long-term benefits of intensive insulin treatment can be hypothesized and increasingly envisioned but remain unproven. These potential benefits must be balanced in each patient against actual risks and costs. With the remaining degree of uncertainty, physicians together with patients should set treatment goals on the basis of their own assessment of the evidence and their best judgment regarding individual patient capabilities and understanding.

BIBLIOGRAPHY

DCCT Research Group: Diabetes Control and Complications Trial (DCCT): results of feasibility study. *Diabetes Care* 10:1–19, 1987

Diabetes Control and Complications Trial: Are continuing studies of metabolic control and microvascular complications in IDDM justified? *N Engl J Med* 318:246–49, 1988

Education

INTRODUCTION

Day-to-day diabetes management is the responsibility of patients and their families. In time, patients must learn to become their own physicians, dietitians, social workers, laboratory technicians, nurses, and pharmacists. As a result, when a patient does not understand what to do, when, and why, an indispensable member of the health-care team is missing. There can be no skimping on thorough patient (and family) education in insulin-dependent (type I) diabetes. This chapter provides guidance in education for the individual health-care provider and can serve as an assessment tool for educators and hospital programs.

GENERAL PRINCIPLES

The goal of diabetes education is to teach the patient how to incorporate diabetes management into daily life and to minimize the patient's dependence on the physician. This helps the patient become *self-sufficient* and *symptom free* through self-reinforced adherence to the medical regimen.

Ideally, a health-care team, consisting of at least a physician, nurse educator, and dietitian, should be involved in patient education. However, many physicians do not have access to a team, in which case other resources can be used. These can include other patients with diabetes and their family members or friends who have successfully lived with the disease and mastered some of its complexities. Local American Diabetes Association (ADA) chapters, hospitals, and visiting nurse associations will know of such resources.

Successful education is a planned, time-requiring process that should take place in an environment both practically and emotionally conducive to learning. A quick interaction on the day of discharge from the hospital is not adequate.

There must be sufficient time to teach, answer questions, and maintain educational materials. However, *large blocks of time are not necessary*. A few minutes spent teaching and reinforcing short lessons, plus close telephone contact to answer "real-life" questions as they arise, can be highly effective. Instructions should be individualized and supported with concise, written explanations. Written information can be obtained from ADA and its local chapters, the National Institutes of Health (NIH), insulin manufacturers, diabetes product manufacturers, and libraries.

INITIAL INTERVIEW AND ASSESSMENT

Education should begin with an in-depth patient assessment as soon as is practical after diagnosis. This crucial interaction can have a life-long influence on the patient's attitudes about diabetes. Its purpose is to obtain information about the patient, to identify areas that will influence adherence, and to build empathy between the patient and educator. *Do not teach—listen* to both the spoken and implied words of the patient and family members. Observe body language, tone of voice, and level of apprehension. Allow time for the patient to express feelings. Allow time for separate interviews with the patient and family if possible. The initial interview and assessment generally requires about 1 hour.

The newly diagnosed patient is likely to be filled with anxieties about death and dying, the use of needles, and the implications of the diagnosis. The educator's highest priority during initial meetings is to encourage the patient to express these fears, to offer reassurance that they are understandable, and to directly explain the degree to which they are either groundless or subject to the patient's own control. Anxieties constitute barriers to learning that must be overcome early if learning is to take place.

Individuals entering an education program who have had diabetes for some time must be assessed for any misinformation they may harbor and for differences between their diabetes knowledge and practice. More generally, the educator should elicit the patient's attitudes toward diabetes and the impact diabetes has made on the patient's and family's life-style.

Areas the initial assessment should address include the following.

■ Health belief system. Does the patient feel in control of his/her life and health? How high a priority was health for that individual before diagnosis of diabetes?

■ Education. The educator should be sensitive to the educational level of the patient and note differences in the language and vocabulary of the patient and relatives. These differences may present problems or be used to an advantage. However, regardless of education level, the most effective language is simple, direct, and free of jargon. Written material should rarely exceed 6th-grade level, which is preferred even by adults with a 12th- grade education and higher.

■ Ethnic background. Traditions, superstititions, and ethnic foods must be taken into account in the management regimen. Repeated contact with specific populations will give the educator experience in identifying factors that may affect diabetes management.

■ Life-style. The patient's daily routines, jobs, hobbies, and weekend activities all affect when and where the patient injects insulin and monitors blood glucose. Shift workers in particular need specific meal and insulin schedules.

■ Eating habits. Eating habits must be assessed before a meal plan can be developed. Meals, especially breakfast, are frequently inadequate or missed altogether, whereas some snacks are enough to constitute a meal.

■ Support system. Family and social factors will influence adherence; for example, family members may provide constant temptation with inadvisable foods. This treatment sabotage, whether unconscious or deliberate, must be recognized and corrected.

"Latch-key" children may be responsible for most of their own health care. In this situation, very precise written management instructions are needed. The patient who lives alone may find management requirements overwhelming and need help from neighbors, Meals on Wheels, religious support groups, or board and care facilities.

The elderly who live alone need additional assessment. Their mental and physical capabilities must be considered, including their ability to prepare meals, self-monitor blood glucose (SMBG) or urine, and measure and inject insulin. Is the patient able to make a telephone call for help? Can this individual treat an insulin reaction? Additional help can be obtained from home-help aides, senior-citizens centers, and hospital support groups.

■ Economic circumstances. For patients on a limited income, costs must be considered. Is the patient employed and insured? If finances are a problem, the physician should be prepared to compromise about the frequency of monitoring, use of a meter, and other costly areas of therapy but should endeavor not to compromise the therapeutic goals. In addition, the dietitian should be alerted that the patient may need special help in food selection and purchasing.

Information about community services for low-income patients can be obtained from a local hospital discharge planner. Additional resources may include state and regional children's services for case management and for covering medical costs; government and/or private job training and placement programs; hospital programs for emergency cash, supplies, and clothes; and local government agencies for board and care. More information on effective teaching is provided in Box 3.

SURVIVAL SKILLS AND CONCEPTS

Survival skills are required by patients to survive outside the hospital. These skills and the basic concepts that underlie them must be learned with 100% accuracy because the patient's life depends on them. It is important for family members, as well as the patient, to understand basic diabetes concepts and skills (Box 4).

Recommended teaching time constitutes a total of approximately 10 hours, which should consist not just of class time but also of phone contact and less

Box 3. Keys to Successful Teaching

Effective teaching will include many of the following strategies.

- Provide ongoing encouragement and emotional support.
- Help overcome anxiety. This may be required to a greater or lesser extent at nearly every session.
- Sequence topics logically from simple to complex, starting with survival skills. Teach less rather than more each session.
- Support oral instructions with concise, specific written material because patients remember <50% of what they are told in the physician's office.
- Have patients solve problems, e.g., "what should you do if you had been getting up to go to the bathroom 3 or 4 times for the past few nights?" "what should you do if you are stuck in a traffic jam without a snack when your insulin is peaking?"

Talking through real-life problems helps the patient learn and alerts the teacher to gaps in patient knowledge.

- Motivate the patient. Young children can be given rewards such as toys. For teens and adults, elicit specific problems that, when solved, will serve as motivators. Give adolescents tips on eating out with a crowd, and offer adults help in integrating work and diabetes schedules. Verbal and written contracts, letters of congratulations, achievement badges, and certificates aid patient adherence.
- Be prepared to compromise. Instead of imposing goals on the patient, negotiate for mutually acceptable goals. For example, instead of monitoring 8 times each day (to obtain a detailed sense of glycemic control), a child might monitor 3–4 times a day for only 2 days a week, e.g., Monday and Thursday the 1st wk, Tuesday and Friday the 2nd wk. Over time, a profile of blood glucose control emerges.
- Keep the treatment regimen simple and realistic. *The patient will adhere to the regimen as long as the required effort does not exceed the perceived benefits.*

formalized communication between the patient and members of the health-care team. More complete information about each topic can be found in the appropriate chapter of the *Guide*.

Insulin Injection

Insulin injection is often so anxiety provoking that it should be taught at the first or second interview and kept separate from lessons on insulin therapy (e.g., how to measure and mix insulin, what insulin does). Some experts recommend that the teacher demonstrate the technique by self-injecting saline. The educator thereby shows the patient that the procedure is not painful. This helps give the patient confidence to try self-injection or to begin by injecting the educator.

Hesitation for more than a few seconds before injection may signal the start of a lasting injection anxiety. The teacher should be prepared to assist by guiding the patient's hand, with a quick push if necessary. Praise is appropriate when the injection is completed. Proficiency is gained only by practice on human skin; oranges are not a satisfactory substitute. Further suggestions on minimizing pain when injecting are listed in Box 5.

As an introduction to self-injection, young and toddler-aged children can be encouraged to inject a favorite stuffed animal while receiving their own injec-

Box 4. Survival Skills

- Insulin injection
- Pathophysiology
- Maintaining balance
- Honeymoon phase
- Meal plan
- Insulin preparations and dosage
- Monitoring
- Hypoglycemia and hyperglycemia
- Sick-day management and DKA
- Supplies and identifications
- Emergency phone numbers

tion. A child's injections should initially be given only by a competent experienced individual.

Toddlers should not be expected to inject themselves regularly but may be allowed to occasionally satisfy their curiosity or as a reward—*never* as a punishment. Children less than 10 to 12 years old can be encouraged to perform their own injections but should not be expected to do so alone unless they are mature enough. By the age of 14, however, most children can be expected, but should not be forced, to perform their own injections under most circumstances.

Box 5. Minimizing Painful Injections

Ways to minimize pain when injecting insulin.

- Inject insulin at room or body temperature.
- Make sure no air bubbles remain in syringe before injecting.
- Wait until topical alcohol has evaporated completely before injecting.
- Keep injection-area muscles limber, not tense, when injecting.
- Penetrate skin quickly.
- Withdraw needle quickly.
- Do not change direction of needle while inserting or withdrawing.
- Do not reuse needles if they are becoming dull.

Pathophysiology

All patients with type I diabetes mellitus must understand the basic mechanism of the disease process. The explanation can be simple, but it must emphasize the life-long daily need to inject insulin that is no longer made by the body.

Maintaining a Balance

People with newly or even previously diagnosed diabetes are often remarkably ignorant of the fact that food and stress raise blood glucose, whereas insulin and activity lower it. These interactions can be illustrated by the educator with the concept of balance. Stable metabolic control can be compared to a balanced scale; then the patient can be shown how various factors may disrupt the balance. It is ideal for an actual scale to be available for the demonstration.

For example, blocks labeled "stress of worry, excitement, or infection" or one representing a piece of cake may be put on one side of the scale. To the other side, blocks representing insulin or exercise may be added. The educator must explain that with sufficient planning and attention to each factor, balance can be maintained most of the time.

Honeymoon (Remission) Phase

The physician should tell patients and their families to anticipate a honeymoon period and should take pains to explain that this remission is invariably temporary. When the honeymoon phase begins, patients and their families should know to watch for hypoglycemia as insulin requirements decline. Because it is not uncommon for patients to mistake a temporary discontinuation of injections for a cure, it is advisable to maintain the usual injection regimen during this time, even if it provides only 1 or 2 units of insulin at each dose.

Meal Plan

Types of food, quantities required, and meal/snack timing need to be taught, with consideration given to the lifestyles and food preferences of the patient and family (see **Nutrition**).

Insulin Preparations and Dosage

The patient must know the name, strength, course of action, dosage, and injection time of the prescribed insulins. The patient must also know to store the insulin between 40 and 85°F.

Accurately measuring insulin and mixing two different types can be difficult skills for some patients and therefore must be assessed periodically, especially when the dosage is changed. The physician or other educator should observe the patient's technique and inspect the bottles in use. Site rotation should also be explained.

Monitoring Technique

Proper self-monitoring technique is crucial to achieve reliable results; therefore, the physician or other educator

Box 6. What School Personnel Need to Know

All school personnel should be aware of the following if they have a child with diabetes in their school.

- Hypoglycemia: signs and symptoms, treatment, and where emergency carbohydrates and snacks are kept. Child may need to be allowed to eat snacks during class and especially before physical education classes or sports.
- Hyperglycemia: child may need to be excused frequently to go to the restroom and water fountain.
- Personal information: this includes a person to call for more information and emergency phone numbers of parent or guardian and physician.

should watch the patient perform self-tests when learning monitoring or later if logged results seem inconsistent with glycohemoglobin levels or other indicators of control. The patient needs written guidelines on interpreting test results, making treatment changes based on test results, and calling for help in response to high glucose and/or ketone levels (see **Monitoring**).

Management of Hypoglycemia

Knowing how to recognize and treat hypoglycemia, including the use of glucagon, is essential for the patient and people close to the patient. For an adult, supervisors and trusted co-workers should learn the symptoms of hypoglycemia and be able to treat it appropriately. For a child, school teachers, lunchroom personnel, school bus drivers, and physical education instructors should be informed. This is best coordinated through the school nurse (Box 6). Prevention and management of hypoglycemia under dangerous circumstances, most commonly driving, should be emphasized (see **Hypoglycemia**).

Management of Hyperglycemia

Patients should be reminded that increased thirst and urination, a dry mouth, bed-wetting, and sometimes weight loss and blurred vision can reflect high blood glucose levels that should be brought to the physician's attention. Parents should be informed of the possibility of deliberate hyperglycemia. Young people sometimes manipulate their insulin doses to test the continued presence of the disease, to seek attention, or to escape from problems at home.

Sick-Day Management and Diabetic Ketoacidosis

The concepts of sick-day management may be difficult for patients and families to understand and practice. *Mismanagement of sick days is a common cause of the preventable problem of diabetic ketoacidosis (DKA).* The medical team must be alert to the patient who has recurring episodes of DKA and must aggressively seek the causes.

Stressful situations, infections, colds, and influenza, which can cause fever, vomiting, or diarrhea, may require intensive management so that diabetes control does not deteriorate to DKA. Short-term illnesses can be frequently managed at home by the patient who follows written guidelines such as those below. When in doubt, the patient should be encouraged to phone the health professional for guidance.

Sick-day rules are a crucial component of survival skills. The following information provides guidelines for the practitioner, and similar guidelines should be given to the patient.

Monitoring

Blood glucose and urinary ketones need to be monitored frequently, often every 2 to 3 hours, and appropriate action should be taken, such as calling the physician if levels are greater than 300 mg/dl by meter or greater than 240 mg/dl by color estimation or levels, stated by the physician's guidelines.

Management of Insulin

Patients must understand that they should *never stop taking insulin*. When insulin is changed, consideration must be given to the patient's sensitivity to insulin, usual treatment regimen, and previous experience with sick-day management. The nature and likely duration of the illness determine whether long-acting insulin should be increased. Supplemental short-acting insulin may need to be given as often as every 3 to 4 hours according to the results of SMBG. A

1-2U / 30-50 mg/dl over 150

broad guideline for an adult is 1 to 2 units of insulin for every 30 to 50 mg/dl that glucose exceeds 150 mg/dl. If hyperglycemia or ketonuria persists, supplemental insulin doses should be doubled.

Fluids and Calories

Light meals eaten six to eight times a day may be tolerated better than the usual food, and semisolids and liquids are often tolerated best during illness. Ten to 20 grams of carbohydrate need to be consumed every 1 to 2 hours. The following contain 15 grams carbohydrate:

- ⅓ cup regular gelatin
- ½ cup vanilla ice cream
- 3 squares graham crackers
- 1 cup cream soup
- ½ cup custard.

If vomiting, diarrhea, or fever is present, small quantities of liquids, taken every 15 to 20 minutes, are recommended (adults may need 8 oz/h). In addition to prevention of dehydration, liquids are needed to compensate for the loss of salt, potassium, and calories. It is important to make clear to the patient that *nondiet* soft drinks and juices are required.

Replacement fluids

- ¾ cup regular ginger ale (~15 g CHO)
- 1 cup Gatorade (~15 g CHO)
- ½ cup Coke (~15 g CHO)
- ½ cup orange juice (~15 g CHO)
- ½ cup broth (~0 g CHO)

The physician should be called when

- more than two insulin supplements are needed;
- vomiting and/or diarrhea are present and the patient has been unable to take fluids for 4 hours or more;
- blood glucose is difficult to control, and/or ketonuria is present; or
- there is no improvement or the illness lasts more than 24 hours.

Supplies for Patients

New patients should be supplied with insulin, syringes, glucagon, cleansing alcohol swabs, lancets or a finger-sticking device, and strips for SMBG and monitoring of urine ketones. They should be instructed on how to obtain more supplies when needed.

Patient Identification

Patients should be urged to wear bracelets that identify them as having type I diabetes mellitus. A wallet card or a necklace can also be beneficial in identifying an unconscious or otherwise impaired diabetic patient.

Emergency Telephone Numbers and Guidelines

The name and telephone number of a main contact with 24-hour availability must be provided for the patient. Directions for emergencies need to be given as well as support personnel telephone numbers and written directions for when to call the physician. Guidelines should include the following:

- blood glucose persistently high (>300 mg/dl by meter, >240 mg/dl by color estimation)
- ketonuria for more than 4 hours
- persistent vomiting
- frequent symptomatic hypoglycemia
- asymptomatic blood glucose levels less than 60 mg/dl.

IN-DEPTH EDUCATION

Ideally, in-depth education should begin shortly after diagnosis, at least within 3 to 4 weeks. Most information should be reviewed annually. Major topics of education are discussed briefly below and in detail in the referenced chapter.

Risks in Pregnancy

Women of childbearing age need to be thoroughly informed about the risks of pregnancy with diabetes. They need to know that conception should occur only *after* meticulous diabetic control has been maintained, ideally for at least 3 months (see **Pregnancy**).

Advice on Exercise

Sedentary patients should be encouraged to gradually increase daily exercise levels. At first, the emphasis should be on increasing activity in daily life, then moving toward an actual exercise program. If exercise is to become routine, it must be perceived as pleasurable.

All patients should be advised of the potential for hypoglycemia during ex-

Table 4. Diabetes Mellitus Patient Education Log*

	DATE LENGTH OF TIME	DATE LENGTH OF TIME	DATE LENGTH OF TIME	DATE LENGTH OF TIME	DATE LENGTH OF TIME	COMMENTS
Pathophysiology						
Definition						
Food blood glucose insulin						
Balance and imbalance						
Reasons for control						
Injection						
Injects self						
Measures doses						
Mixes 2 insulins						
Site rotation						
Medication schedule						
Insulin						
Action of prescribed insulins						
Identifies insulins						
Storage						
Monitoring of blood glucose						
Method						
Reads results						
Records results						
Interprets results						
Adjusts insulin						
When to test						
Ketonuria						
Method						
Reads results						
Records results						
Interpretation						
When to test						
Patient identification	Instructor's name/Date	Instructor's name/Date	Instructor's name/Date	Instructor's name/Date	Instructor's name/Date	

*Codes: I, instructed; N, does not understand; S, some understanding, needs reinforcement, assistance; R, reviewed; C, competent; OI, incapable, needs outside assistance.

ercise. This applies particularly to patients involved in intensive exercise or competitive games (see **Exercise**).

Chronic Complications

At the time of diagnosis, the patient and the family have enough emotionally trying information to absorb without having to cope with news that diabetes can cause long-term debilitating complications. However, many teenagers and adults will already be aware of the possibility of complications. If a patient asks about complications or gives the clinician a sense that this is a concern, the subject should be discussed honestly and openly. This is especially important if the patient seems misinformed.

Regardless of how soon after diagnosis the subject of complications is raised, the patient needs a clear understanding of what is known and unknown about the relationship between blood glucose control and complications (see **Philosophy and Goals**). The patient should also be informed about the importance of controlling risk factors, e.g., blood fats, obesity, smoking, and hypertension, because these interact with diabetes to increase the risks of complications.

The possibility of preventing or delaying long-term complications is a legitimate motivation for adhering to a diabetes treatment plan. However, the prospect of complications should not be used as a scare tactic to improve adherence; this strategy yields short-lived results at best and can anger the patient.

Eye Care

The patient needs to have annual eye examinations after 5 years of diabetes (this need not be done before puberty). The patient should call the physician if any of the following symptoms appear:

- changes in vision
- floating spots on front of eyes
- difficulty seeing in the dark
- colored rings or halos around lights
- pressure or pain in the eyes
- hypersensitivity to light.

Foot Care

Foot-care skills are best taught by demonstrating on one foot, with the patient giving a return demonstration on the other. When the patient is incapable of caring adequately for his/her feet, a responsible relative or friend must be taught. The rules for care and guidelines for identifying problem areas need to be provided in an easy-to-read written format. The patient should call the physician regarding any of the following: ingrown toenails; skin abrasions that are not healing; red, swollen, sore areas; discoloration; and/or infections.

Hygiene Guidelines

The principles of good hygiene need to be reiterated to the diabetic patient, who is at an increased risk for infection when hyperglycemic. Perineal care needs to be discussed in detail with all female patients.

Career and Job Placement

Although nearly every career is open to diabetic patients, certain positions may be poor choices. Jobs that involve long periods between meals or highly erratic schedules place special demands on the diabetes regimen. Career suggestions, if solicited, should advise against jobs that require operating dangerous machinery.

Travel Guidelines

Insulin and diabetes supplies sufficient for the whole trip need to be carried with the patient and not in consigned baggage to prevent loss or temperature extremes. Information on physicians in foreign countries, taking snack foods when meals are delayed, and crossing time zones should be discussed.

Driving a Motor Vehicle

Any patient who drives should be taught to self-monitor blood glucose and adjust food intake and insulin dose before starting the car if the last meal was eaten more than 3 hours earlier or if the journey will be long. If a reaction starts on the road, the driver must pull over, stop the car, treat the reaction, and continue only when safe. Along with wearing a diabetes identification bracelet, insulin-requiring drivers must always carry candy, Lifesavers, or a can of sugar-containing soft drink to treat a reaction.

EVALUATING AND DOCUMENTING TEACHING

The patient's learning must be evaluated both over the short and long term by a combination of verbal repetition, written questionnaire, and return demonstration with 100% accuracy for basic skills including SMBG and meal-planning techniques. This evaluation is imperative for the patient and reveals the effectiveness of the teacher.

Physicians should keep teaching records that show, by measurable criteria, what patients have learned and how well they have learned it (Table 4). This record aids in the exchange of information and the coordination of teaching by all team members and supplies necessary information to health insurance companies.

CONCLUSION

Diabetes education is a long and complex process. The magnitude of the lifestyle changes and the amount of effort involved in adhering to the treatment regimen cannot be fully appreciated by health-care providers who do not have diabetes. Understanding and practicing the complexities of living with diabetes would increase empathy and enhance the skills of health-care providers.

BIBLIOGRAPHY

American Diabetes Association: *Goals for Diabetes Education.* Alexandria, VA, Am. Diabetes Assoc., 1987

Etzwiler D: Patient education and management: a team approach. In *Diabetes Mellitus, Theory and Practice.* 3rd ed., New York, Medical Examination Publishers, 1983, p. 1063–69

Kilo C: Educating the diabetic patient. In *Science and Medicine.* New York, Pfizer, 1982

National Diabetes Advisory Board: National standards for diabetes patient education programs. *Diabetes Care* 7:xxxi–xv, 1984

Routine Management: Tools

Highlights
Routine Management: Tools

INSULIN TREATMENT

Patients with type I diabetes are dependent on insulin to survive.

Insulin preparations are classified by species (beef, pork, and human) and duration of action (short, intermediate, and long acting) (Table 5, p. 32).

Highly purified animal or human insulin is associated with fewer insulin antibodies, less insulin allergy, and less lipoatrophy at the injection site.

The insulin regimen will be shaped to the needs of the individual patient. **Therapy adjustments should be based on actual glycemic values** obtained from patient self-monitoring of blood glucose (SMBG) rather than on "textbook" predictions of insulin action.

Single-injection regimens are usually inadequate in treating type I diabetes. Twice-daily insulin injections should be started as soon as possible after diagnosis to facilitate acceptance by patient and family. The two doses may consist of

- intermediate-acting insulin alone,
- a fixed or flexible split-mixed regimen of two doses of mixed short- and intermediate-acting insulin,
- three or more injections per day, or
- insulin infusion pump therapy.

Insulin needs may fluctuate during the first weeks or months of treatment. If a honeymoon phase occurs, insulin dose must be appropriately reduced, occasionally to as little as 0.1 $U \cdot kg^{-1} \cdot day^{-1}$.

Common problems associated with insulin therapy are detailed on pages 36–38.

Regimens employing insulin algorithms place more demands on both patient and physician than a fixed course of treatment. **All forms of intensive therapy require very high degrees of commitment on the part of the patient, the family, and the health-care team.**

Completely normal blood glucose values are extremely difficult to obtain except under rigorous research conditions.

Instructions for intensifying insulin therapy are contained in Box 9, page 38.

Continuous subcutaneous insulin infusion (p. 39) is a particularly demanding form of therapy, with its physical, psychological, financial, and practical day-by-day burdens. Problems may also be associated with the pump itself (p. 40).

MONITORING

Patients can only manage their diabetes effectively and safely if they are able to perform self-monitoring.

Monitoring allows objective goals for therapy and a means to measure the efficacy of changes in therapy.

Urine glucose testing (p. 41) is easy and inexpensive. However, urine tests cannot provide information about blood glucose in the acceptable or hypoglycemic range. Urine tests serve as integrators, averaging the ups and downs of blood glucose levels.

Self-monitoring of blood glucose (SMBG) (p. 41) is the only monitoring method that allows

- detection and prevention of hypoglycemia and
- adjustment of insulin, diet, and exercise to achieve target blood glucose levels.

Two SMBG measurements a day, every day, usually provide sufficient information to adjust insulin and diet. Additional tests are advisable when exercising, on sick days, or when schedule has changed (Box 10, p. 43).

Common causes of errors are presented on page 44. They include an inadequate drop of blood on the strip, poor technique in removing the blood from the strip, and inaccurate timing.

Urine testing is the only practical way to detect ketones (acetone). **All patients must test urine for ketones during illness.**

A properly performed glycosylated hemoglobin assay provides the best available index of chronic glucose levels. It is highly reliable and virtually tamperproof.

NUTRITION

The meal plan for type I diabetes is a guideline for consistency in food intake to aid in diabetes control.

Calories should be prescribed to achieve and maintain a desirable body weight (p. 46). Baseline calorie needs take into account age, height, weight, need for weight loss or gain, and usual activity and/or exercise patterns.

Recommendations for the nutrient content, including carbohydrate, protein, and fat, are described on pages 46–49. They are similar to recommendations for nondiabetic people developed by other major health organizations.

Up to 55 to 60% of total calories can be consumed as carbohydrates, preferably in the form of unrefined high-fiber complex carbohydrate. Higher-fiber foods should be introduced gradually. In select individuals, sucrose and other refined sugars may be acceptable on occasion.

For most adults and children, protein should contribute about 15 to 20% of total calories. Fat should contribute less than 30% of total calories. Any reduction in fat should be considered a positive step.

Additional nutrition considerations are outlined on pages 49–52.

The registered dietitian is the preferred professional for managing nutrition needs of patients with type I diabetes.

EXERCISE

A specific exercise program should be part of the treatment plan for all patients with type I diabetes.

Physiological responses to exercise in nondiabetic people and in patients with type I diabetes are described in Box 12, page 55. For the type I patient, **plasma insulin levels during and after exercise are critical determinants of response.**

Potential benefits of exercise are explained on page 54. Intense exercise ameliorates cardiovascular risk factors. Mild, moderate, and intense exercise may

- improve glycemic control,
- aid in weight control, and
- heighten sense of well-being.

Potential risks of exercise include destabilization of metabolic control, e.g.,

- hypoglycemia during or after exercise (most likely with sporadic exercise) and
- hyperglycemia to the point of ketoacidosis (if diabetes is controlled at a minimal level or blood glucose is high before beginning activity). Other risks of exercise are described on page 56.

A preexercise medical evaluation (p. 56) **should be performed regardless of the patient's age.**

Exercise should be prescribed with caution in patients with

- minimally controlled blood glucose;
- cardiovascular disease, neuropathy, or proliferative retinopathy; or
- hypoglycemic unawareness.

Guidelines for safe exercise are addressed in Box 14, page 56. They include

- monitoring blood glucose and taking appropriate action,
- altering food or insulin if needed,
- carrying short-acting carbohydrate and identification, and
- monitoring intensity of exercise.

Insulin Treatment

INTRODUCTION

Insulin-dependent (type I) diabetes mellitus is characterized by a near-absolute deficiency in endogenous insulin secretion. Affected patients are dependent on insulin to survive for the duration of their lives. Insulin injections are the mainstay of treatment and must be individualized for each patient.

INSULIN PREPARATIONS

Insulin preparations are generally classified by species (beef, pork, and human) and duration of action (short, intermediate, and long acting). Many insulin preparations are available; as a practical matter, health professionals should familiarize themselves with several of them and learn to use them rationally (Tables 5 and 6).

Species and Purity

Standard (conventionally purified) preparations of beef and/or pork insulin contain significant impurities but much less than in previous years. However, these preparations are no longer produced in the United States. Highly purified insulins of animal origin are now standard and contain less than 10 parts per million of impurities and are associated with a reduced incidence of insulin antibodies, less insulin allergy, and less lipoatrophy at the injection site than previous preparations. Human insulin prepared by recombinant DNA techniques or by chemical modification of animal insulin (semisynthetic) is also available and may be even more pure.

As a foreign protein, animal insulin may be antigenic. Beef insulin differs from the human molecule by two amino acids, making it more antigenic than pork, which differs by only one amino acid. Human insulin, available only in highly purified form, is the least antigenic insulin on the market.

A theoretical advantage of human insulin over pure pork insulin, or of pure pork over standard beef or combinations of beef and pork, is that minimizing or avoiding antibody production may improve blood glucose control. Some researchers believe that circulating antibodies may bind and subsequently release insulin, leading to unpredictable levels of the hormone. If this is the case, less antigenic preparations should improve glycemic stability. The clinician should be aware that human insulin may *act quicker, peak earlier, and last a shorter time than animal insulins.* Lipoatrophy at the injection site, probably related to impurities, may be prevented with either human or pure pork preparations.

It is still unclear whether all patients using animal insulins should change to pure pork or human insulin. Generally, patients started on one type of insulin should be maintained on it as long as they are doing well. In the future, human insulin will probably replace all other currently available types.

Duration of Action

Although insulins are classified into short-, intermediate-, and long-acting preparations, actual insulin effects do not always coincide with such simple descriptions. For example, local subcutaneous tissue conditions not clearly understood may cause rates of absorption to vary by up to 25% from day to day in any one patient. In light of the many other variables influencing insulin pharmacokinetics, the clinician is cautioned against relying too heavily on textbook descriptions of insulin action. Health professionals should base therapy adjustments on actual glycemic values obtained from the patient's self-monitoring of blood glucose (SMBG).

Any change in the dose of intermediate-acting (NPH or lente) insulin requires a 2- to 5-day observation before further dose adjustment because of the relatively slow absorption of these insulins and because of day-to-day variability in food, activity, and stress. An even longer period of observation is needed for long-acting preparations.

The use of SMBG to map out a profile of blood glucose values is invaluable in assisting the physician, patient, and health-care team with therapy. Particularly when initiating or intensifying insulin therapy or when seeking the cause of hypoglycemia or hyperglycemia,

Table 5. Insulins Sold in the United States

PRODUCT	MANUFACTURER	STRENGTH
Short-acting (usual onset 0.5–2.0 h; usual duration 3–6 h)		
Human		
Humulin regular	Lilly	U-100
Humulin BR (only external insulin pumps)	Lilly	U-100
Novolin R (regular, formerly Actrapid human)	Squibb-Novo	U-100
Velosulin human (regular)	Nordisk-USA	U-100
Novolin R Penfill (regular)	Squibb-Novo	U-100
Beef		
Iletin II regular	Lilly	U-100
Semilente	Squibb-Novo	U-100
Pork		
Iletin II regular	Lilly	U-100, U-500
Purified pork R (regular, formerly Actrapid)	Squibb-Novo	U-100
Velosulin (regular)	Nordisk-USA	U-100
Purified pork S (semilente, formerly Semitard)	Squibb-Novo	U-100
Regular	Squibb-Novo	U-100
Beef/Pork		
Iletin I (regular)	Lilly	U-40, U-100
Iletin I (Semilente)	Lilly	U-40, U-100
Intermediate acting (usual onset 3–6 h; usual duration 12–20 h)		
Human		
Humulin L	Lilly	U-100
Humulin NPH	Lilly	U-100
Insulatard human NPH	Nordisk-USA	U-100
Novolin L (lente, formerly Monotard human)	Squibb-Novo	U-100
Novolin N (NPH)	Squibb-Novo	U-100
Beef		
Iletin II Lente	Lilly	U-100
Iletin II NPH	Lilly	U-100
NPH	Squibb-Novo	U-100
Pork		
Iletin II Lente	Lilly	U-100
Iletin II NPH	Lilly	U-100
Insulatard NPH	Nordisk-USA	U-100
Purified pork lente (formerly Monotard)	Squibb-Novo	U-100
Purified pork N (NPH, formerly Protaphane)	Squibb-Novo	U-100
Beef/pork		
Iletin I Lente	Lilly	U-40, U-100
Iletin I NPH	Lilly	U-40, U-100
Long acting (usual onset 6–12 h; usual duration 18–36 h)		
Human		
Humulin U (Ultralente)	Lilly	U-100
Beef		
Iletin II PZI	Lilly	U-100
Purified beef U (ultralente, formerly Ultratard)	Squibb-Novo	U-100
Ultralente	Squibb-Novo	U-100
Beef/pork		
Iletin I PZI	Lilly	U-40, U-100
Iletin I Ultralente	Lilly	U-40, U-100
Premixed combinations		
Human		
Novolin 70/30	Squibb-Novo	U-100
Pork		
Mixtard (30% regular, 70% NPH)	Nordisk-USA	U-100

Table 6. Insulins by Relative Comparative Action Curves

INSULIN	ONSET (h)	PEAK (h)	USUAL EFFECTIVE DURATION (h)	USUAL MAXIMUM DURATION (h)
Animal				
Regular	0.5–2.0	3–4	4–6	6–8
NPH	4–6	8–14	16–20	20–24
Lente	4–6	8–14	16–20	20–24
Ultralente	8–14	Minimal	24–36	24–36
Human				
Regular	0.5–1.0	2–3	3–6	4–6
NPH	2–4	4–10	10–16	14–18
Lente	3–4	4–12	12–18	16–20
Ultralente	6–10	?	18–20	20–30

blood glucose should be measured before and after meals and several times during the night. Routine frequency of monitoring should be based on mutually defined goals described in **Philosophy and Goals.**

Mixing Insulins

The action-prolonging substances in intermediate- or long-acting insulin (NPH, lente, and ultralente) can sometimes affect the onset, peak, and duration of effectiveness of short-acting insulin in a mixture. Generally, the longer the contact time between the two types of insulin and the larger the proportion of intermediate- or longer-acting insulin in the mixture, the less rapid absorption of the short-acting insulin. Therefore, blood glucose levels fall at a slower rate, but the effect lasts longer. NPH may have a less pronounced effect on comixed regular insulin than does the lente series of insulins.

Mixing regular insulin with NPH in the same syringe is an accepted and convenient way to produce differently timed pharmacologic actions with a single injection. Similarly, semilente can be mixed with lente to improve the short-acting effect. (Lente is a mixture of 70% ultralente and 30% semilente.) Stable premixtures of intermediate- and short-acting insulin in fixed proportion (e.g., 70% NPH/30% regular) are also commercially available. Premixed insulins are not suitable when daily variation in the dose of short-acting insulin is required.

INSULIN REGIMENS

Normal insulin secretion is characterized by continuous basal release, with superimposed bursts of additional insulin precisely integrated to the rise in blood glucose after food intake. Additionally, insulin is secreted into the portal vein and thus goes to the liver before entering the general circulation. Ideally, exogenous insulin treatment regimens would mimic all aspects of this pattern. However, this is not clinically possible; therefore, insulin treatment regimens represent varying degrees of compromise.

One-Injection Regimens

Too often, patients with type I diabetes are treated with a single morning injection of intermediate-acting insulin, alone or in combination with short-acting insulin. Whether such a regimen is adopted at the request of the patient or because the physician believes that patients will not accept more than one injection a day, *it is almost always inadequate.* In most patients, a morning injection of NPH or lente insulin is insufficient to prevent hyperglycemia during the night and before breakfast the next morning.

Two-Injection Regimens

Most diabetologists believe that patients with type I diabetes need a *minimum* of two injections per day to obtain sufficient insulin through the waking hours as well as adequate (although lowered) overnight insulin. A typical twice-daily insulin prescription provides a total daily dose of 0.6 to 1.0 $U \cdot kg^{-1} \cdot day^{-1}$,* with two-thirds given in the morning before breakfast and one-third given before supper (Figure 3*A*).

The two doses may consist of intermediate-acting insulin alone. However, a split-mixed regimen, with two doses of mixed short- and intermediate-acting insulins, may provide better control. A third alternative is a split-mixed regimen where, instead of using fixed doses, the patient adjusts the amount of short-acting insulin in response to SMBG results and an algorithm.

Figure 3. Various Insulin-Delivery Schemes (Before Individualizing for Meal Plan, Exercise, and Life-Style)

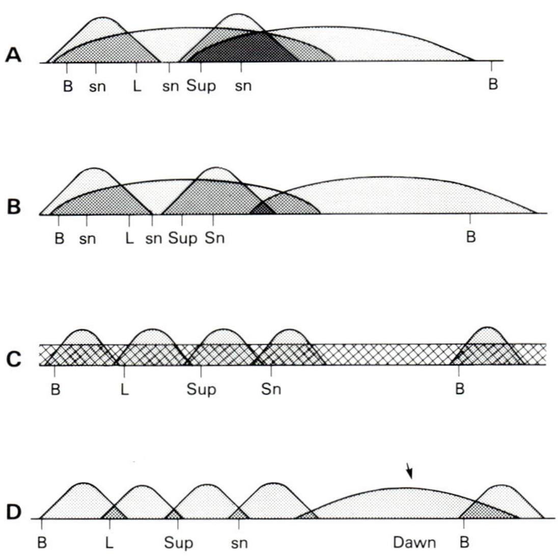

A: standard twice-daily insulin regimen (e.g., intermediate and short acting). *B*: 3-times-daily insulin regimen, suggested for patients with early-morning hypoglycemia followed by rebound hyperglycemia or for patients with early-morning hyperglycemia (dawn phenomenon). *C*: multidose insulin regimen; 4 injections/day (short-acting insulin before meals and long-acting at bedtime). *D*: alternative multidose regimen consisting of 5 injections (short-acting insulin premeal and intermediate-acting insulin at bedtime). *Shaded areas* illustrate overlap between insulin peaks.

*$U \cdot kg^{-1} \cdot day^{-1}$ is often written U/(kg · day) or U/kg/day.

Other Insulin Regimens

Alternative insulin delivery regimens of increasing sophistication include the following.

Three injections a day (TID) is a common variation if a two-injection regimen, with mixed doses before breakfast and supper, fails to deliver sufficient insulin to prevent fasting hyperglycemia. Typically, the 1700 to 1800 h dose of short-acting insulin is retained to counterbalance the glycemic effects of the evening meal, but the intermediate portion of that injection is delayed until bedtime (Figure 3*B*).

Multidose insulin (MDI) therapy features three or four injections of short-acting insulin preceding meals coupled with longer-acting preparations that mimic basal insulin secretion. The regimen may consist of premeal short-acting insulin plus ultralente once or twice a day or premeal regular insulin with bedtime lente or NPH (Figure 3, *C* and *D*).

Continuous subcutaneous insulin infusion (CSII), or insulin pump therapy, delivers basal short-acting insulin and permits the patient to administer bursts of insulin before meals (it looks similar to Figure 3*C*). MDI and CSII are used in intensified treatment protocols aimed at near normalization of blood glucose results.

All of these options are extremely variable and should be individualized according to meal plan, exercise, and life-style requirements. SMBG should be used frequently to profile glycemic values and to adjust therapy. Additionally, it is paramount that all treatment goals be mutually agreed on by the patient and the health-care team.

TREATING NEWLY DIAGNOSED PATIENTS

Diagnosis and Stabilization

At diagnosis, initial objectives of therapy are eliminating symptomatic hyperglycemia (and concomitant fluid and electrolyte imbalance) while avoiding hypoglycemia; therefore, glycemic targets should be approached gradually. Treatment should begin with approximately 0.5 $U \cdot kg^{-1} \cdot day^{-1}$. However, during the first few days of therapy, this amount can be expected to rise to an average of 1 $U \cdot kg^{-1} \cdot day^{-1}$, because most patients are relatively insulin resistant at this time.

Regimen

Twice-daily insulin, used soon after diagnosis and stabilization of acute metabolic abnormalities, usually prevents excessive hyperglycemia and minimizes hypoglycemia. The total daily insulin dose is usually divided, with approximately 50 to 70% administered in the morning before breakfast and the other 30 to 50% administered either before supper or at bedtime.

Although once-daily insulin may suffice for a short time in patients who retain some beta-cell function, psychological acceptance of two injections daily is easier for both patient and family if it is introduced as soon as possible after diagnosis, even if glycemic control could be adequate on one injection per day.

Insulin Dose

Generally, adults and children require less insulin than adolescents. For example, a newly diagnosed 5-year-old child weighing 22 kilograms may need only 0.4 to 0.8 $U \cdot kg^{-1} \cdot day^{-1}$. Adolescent doses are generally but not always larger. A 15-year-old weighing 50 kilograms might start with 1.0 $U \cdot kg^{-1} \cdot day^{-1}$ but require as much as 50% more or less than that amount.

Note that new patients may experience some problems resembling insulin allergy that are actually related to injection technique (see p. 40).

Honeymoon Phase: Lower Insulin Requirements

Within weeks after diagnosis there may be some recovery of beta-cell function, and consequently, exogenous insulin requirements often decrease for a period of weeks to months. This "honeymoon" or "remission" phase of type I diabetes is often marked by the appearance of recurrent hypoglycemic episodes. A honeymoon phase occurs less frequently in children less than 2 years old; it is more common in the late teenage years and in adults.

If a honeymoon phase occurs, insulin dosage must be appropriately reduced, occasionally to as little as 0.1 $U \cdot kg^{-1} \cdot day^{-1}$. Not all patients exhibit a profound honeymoon phase, but some period of stability in blood glucose levels is common, with insulin requirements at 0.2 to 0.5 $U \cdot kg^{-1} \cdot day^{-1}$. (For more on the honeymoon period, see **Pathogenesis,** p. 12.)

Developing a Long-Term Regimen

Eventually, as beta-cell function decreases over the first 6 to 18 months of therapy, insulin requirements rise to an average of 0.6 to 0.8 $U \cdot kg^{-1} \cdot day^{-1}$. Teenagers may need as much as 1.0 to 1.5 $U \cdot kg^{-1} \cdot day^{-1}$ during the rapid growth spurt associated with puberty but then return to lower preadolescent insulin requirements when puberty is completed. Dose requirements for pregnant type I patients vary with gestational duration and are discussed in detail in **Pregnancy,** p. 79.

A regular rotation of insulin injection sights involving upper arm, thigh, buttocks, and abdominal wall should be used in all subcutaneous insulin treatment regimens. Regular rotation diminishes the likelihood of lipodystrophic changes and/or fibrosis at any one sight and, hence, facilitates absorption. In preadolescent children, injection into the abdominal wall may be painful and therefore may be omitted.

During the months of rapid change, the patient and physician should develop an insulin regimen that helps achieve levels of glycemia and life-style flexibility that they consider desirable and achievable. For many patients, a regimen of two daily doses of a fixed proportion of intermediate- and short-acting insulin will satisfy these needs.

Generally, the correctness of the morning short-acting insulin is judged by the postbreakfast and/or prelunch blood glucose level. Likewise, the correctness of the evening portion of short-acting insulin is judged by the postsupper or bedtime blood glucose level. The correctness of the morning intermediate-acting insulin is judged by the midafternoon blood glucose level, whereas the evening dose of intermediate-acting insulin is judged by the blood glucose level in the early hours of the morning (0200–0700 h).

Box 7. Evaluating Blood Glucose Control: Factors to Consider

- Increase frequency of SMBG for 2–3 days; patient should measure blood glucose 6–8 times a day (fasting, pre- and postprandial, and bedtime values).

Blood glucose values of 80 mg/dl (fasting) to 140 mg/dl (postprandial) may be considered ideal; values between 70 and 200 mg/dl are acceptable; and values <60 or >240 mg/dl are generally considered unacceptable.

- With patient, identify the probable cause of high or low blood glucose values; consider the following:
  - Exercise: forgotten, "burst," after long inactivity, prolonged
  - Snacks: forgotten, concealed, omitted, too small or large
  - Meals: advanced or delayed, time between injection of short-acting insulin and meal, day-to-day consistency in meal timing and/or size
  - Emotional upset: forgotten, considered unimportant
  - Alcohol or drugs
  - Illness or infection
  - Technique of insulin injection: into exercising limb or hypertrophied tissue, variation in depth, ability to draw up correct dose, short- and long-acting insulins reversed, day-to-day variability in timing of intermediate-acting injection
- Technique of SMBG: timing, pad covered, meter readable, expired strips
- Insulin reactions: treatment of undocumented, overtreatment, hypoglycemic unawareness
- Deliberate nonadherence to regimen: insulin omission to lose weight, snacking, emotional problem or eating disorder
- Note recurring glycemic patterns; factors such as the following may be operative:
- Fasting hyperglycemia: single-injection regimen/dawn phenomenon, rebound hyperglycemia
- Late-afternoon hypoglycemia: single-injection regimen
- Overnight hypoglycemia: intermediate-acting insulin dose too large or injected too early
- Erratic glycemic patterns may also result from overinsulinization, antibody binding of insulin, or gastrointestinal motility disorders
- Alter therapy appropriately (see Box 8).

ONGOING THERAPY: COMMON PROBLEMS

Problems in insulin therapy will arise regardless of the insulin regimen, and they must be addressed. Detecting and eliminating patterns of hypoglycemia and hyperglycemia is the bread and butter of caring for the patient with diabetes. This is as true for the individual with diabetes of several years' duration as for the newly diagnosed patient.

One-Injection Regimens

Patients on one-injection regimens commonly experience afternoon or evening hypoglycemia often in combination with nocturnal hyperglycemia. Frequently, a major improvement in glycemic control will result from a change to one of the two-injection regimens described above.

Some patients refuse to take more than one injection a day. Clinical and biochemical goals should always be reviewed with these patients, and sometimes better understanding of the reasons for changing to more than a single morning injection leads to acceptance (see **Philosophy and Goals,** p. 17). Among some adolescents and a few adults, a once-daily regimen, which usually results in only a minimal level of treatment, may be the only outcome achievable without alienating the patient.

Other Issues

Recurrent moderate or severe hypoglycemic reactions signal the need for evaluation of the insulin regimen, eating patterns, and other life-style factors (e.g., alcohol) (see **Hypoglycemia,** Box 21). Exceptionally low glycosylated hemoglobin levels may identify patients at risk for moderate and/or severe hypoglycemia. Some patients have diminished symptoms of impending hypoglycemia and thus suffer from recurrent hypoglycemic reactions and/or hypoglycemic seizures. In patients with such "hypoglycemic unawareness," blood glucose targets must be raised.

Fasting hyperglycemia may occur in conjunction with *high or low* blood glucose values. If SMBG between 0200 and 0400 h reveals nocturnal hypoglycemia, rebound hyperglycemia (Somogyi phenomenon) may be operative (see **Hypoglycemia,** p. 74) and a lowering of evening intermediate-acting insulin called for. However, if no nocturnal hypoglycemia can be documented, inadequate insulin from 0400 to 0900 h (sometimes called the dawn phenomenon) may be causative. This should be addressed with either an increase in presupper insulin or a change to a bedtime injection schedule.

Inconsistencies of food intake and/or activity, often associated with psychosocial factors, can be causes of unacceptable day-to-day glucose control or glycosylated hemoglobin levels.

Other factors that may contribute to glycemic irregularities are listed in Box 7, and a representative case is described in Box 8. Other problems of insulin therapy, including changes in insulin absorption or sensitivity, surgery, hypoglycemia, and insulin allergy are discussed in subsequent parts of this chapter or in other chapters of the *Guide* (see Index).

Once sources of hypoglycemia and hyperglycemia have been eliminated, further efforts to tighten control may require more intensified insulin-delivery protocols than are achievable with fixed twice-daily regimens.

MORE INTENSIFIED INSULIN REGIMENS

Tightening a Split-Mixed Regimen: Use of Algorithms

Insulin algorithms are protocols for adjusting the dose of insulin several times

Box 8. Case Study: SMBG to Improve Therapy

Eight-year-old Janine weighs 22 kg and is on a split-mixed regimen of human insulin: 3 regular plus 12 lente prebreakfast and 1 regular plus 3 lente presupper. Recently, she has had several hypoglycemic convulsions between 0200 and 0330 h, despite increases in her bedtime snack. Sometimes, but not always, the convulsions occur after an afternoon soccer game. A blood glucose profile reveals the following.

Breakfast		Lunch			Snack		
Before	After	Before	After	Supper	Bedtime	0200 h	0400 h
108	248	81	165	84	219	36	52
188	312	242	118	97	145	78	42

Suggested Treatment

Overnight hypoglycemia probably results from middle-of-the-night peaking of lente insulin, sometimes superimposed on the effects of late-afternoon activity. Verify that adherence is not an issue and that Janine's bedtime snack is large enough to balance increased exercise.

Divide the presupper insulin dose to provide 1–2 U regular insulin alone before supper (unless blood glucose is controlled adequately by morning lente plus afternoon activity). Give lente alone at bedtime to delay peak effect toward 0700–0800 h rather than 0100–0300 h. Reduce the next morning's regular insulin to 1–2 units, because bedtime lente insulin will be available to counter the postbreakfast glycemic rise. Morning lente insulin may occasionally be increased a few units as well, based on pre- and postsupper blood glucose.

Recheck middle-of-the-night values to ensure they are >70 mg/dl, and reemphasize the need for extra calories or less insulin on the days Janine plays soccer.

Box 9. Steps to Intensifying Therapy

- Obtain baseline blood glucose profile, glycosylated hemoglobin, and fasting lipids as well as baseline ophthalmologic and renal parameters, for example.
- If patient is on 1-injection regimen, start split-mixed short-acting plus intermediate-acting insulin twice daily.
- Adjust meals and snacks to optimize timing, calories, and source of carbohydrate.
- Instruct patient to perform SMBG 4 times daily (prebreakfast, prelunch, presupper, and prebedtime) and to keep detailed written daily records. Verify accuracy of technique by direct observation.
- Instruct patient to identify probable cause of high or low glucose values (e.g., overeating, late meal, skipped snack, excess activity, illness).
- Schedule office visits more frequently for detailed discussion and review of SMBG results, feedback from staff, and help with problem solving.
- Increase SMBG to include postprandial periods and several measurements during the night. Examine SMBG pattern for subtle asymptomatic hypoglycemia or nocturnal hypoglycemia (with or without subsequent hyperglycemia) as well as waning prebreakfast insulin effect.
- Adjust short-acting insulin doses according to individually constructed algorithms. All doses must be individualized for each patient. Use postprandial SMBG to recheck algorithm efficacy for correcting high or low glucose values toward 100 mg/dl.
- Change from twice-daily insulin-delivery regimen to 3- to 4-times-daily insulin.
- Consider changing to alternative insulin type or species to better match individual requirements.
- Consider alternative delivery device or apparatus to promote adherence.
- If goals remain unmet, verify that dietary and SMBG adherence and contact with staff are optimal. If these are problems, redefine objectives to improve adherence. Use of an insulin pump is contraindicated if poor adherence is documented.
- If goals are satisfied, consider alternative ways to deliver insulin via available devices, e.g., an insulin pump, injections without needles (jet injection devices), indwelling subcutaneous catheters, prefilled cartridge injectors.

a day based on regularly checked blood glucose levels. They also allow patients to adjust insulin dose in relation to amount and composition of food and exercise. Although flexible, such regimens tend to place more demands on both patient and physician than a fixed course of treatment. Box 9 presents a step-by-step approach to improving and intensifying therapy.

The physician develops an algorithm for the patient from premeal blood glucose determinations. A change of 1 to 2 units of short-acting insulin is prescribed for every 40- to 50-mg/dl increment (or decrement) in blood glucose level from a defined blood glucose target. This typical 1- to 2-unit change is modified for individual patients based on the total dosage each day and sensitivity to short-acting insulin. Carbohydrate algorithms are also available, but their use is not as well established.

Initial Goals

Initial goals of glycemic improvement programs include approaching normal blood glucose levels without excessive or severe hypoglycemia. Therefore, a goal for preprandial blood glucose levels may start at 150 to 200 mg/dl but gradually decrease toward 100 mg/dl. Ideal normal premeal values of 70 to 120 mg/dl with 1- to 2-hour postprandial values of less than 180 mg/dl and a return to middle-of-the-night values in the range of 70 to 120 mg/dl are *extremely difficult* to obtain except under rigorous research conditions.

The ability of insulin algorithms to improve control is predicated on (1) reasonable and consistent adherence to meal plans, (2) regular timing and adjustment of insulin based on SMBG, and (3) a regular pattern of activity or exercise. Algorithms may be used to correct for a given value or to adjust insulin dose in anticipation of any blood glucose–altering factors, e.g., increased sugar intake, most intercurrent infections, or decreased physical activity.

Once fasting and premeal values are in line with mutually defined goals, postprandial and middle-of-the-night SMBG can be performed periodically to double-check glycemic excursions and to perfect the treatment regimen. The patient whose average blood glucose value improves but who has recurrent episodes of moderate or severe hypoglycemia is, by definition, still not in good control. *SMBG is as important for detecting and avoiding hypoglycemia as for identifying hyperglycemia.*

Ongoing Goals

Health-care providers must continue to modify expectations as appropriate for the specific patient and family circumstances.

Intensive Insulin Therapy: MDI and CSII

Because of the possibility that more intensive blood glucose control may prevent or decrease late vascular complications, MDI regimens or pump therapy may be an option for some patients. Intensive therapy must be approached with knowledge and caution. *All forms of intensive therapy require very high degrees of commitment on the part of the patient, the family, and the health-care team.* Exceptional dedication, knowledge, and time commitments are the rule. Demands of CSII are particularly stringent, requiring even more rigorous adherence to SMBG and other aspects of management and careful coordination by a team of experienced professionals. Because of the complexity of this problem, patients who are intent on achieving optimal glycemic control are best managed with an experienced team that includes a nurse trained in diabetes control, a diabetologist (or pediatric diabetologist), dietitian, and psychosocial counselor.

The following is an initial approximation of insulin requirements. (For the depth of detail needed to implement intensive therapy, including pump therapy, see Bibliography.)

Basal Insulin Requirements

Basal insulin requirements using either ultralente insulin with MDI or basal regular insulin with CSII are approximately 50% of the patient's previous total daily dose. The remaining 50% is given as short-acting insulin delivered just before meals and/or snacks either by syringe, through an in situ catheter or pressure injector, or by an insulin pump pulse. A typical starting distribution would be 20% of the total daily dose as a short-acting insulin pulse to cover breakfast, 10% to cover lunch, 15% to cover supper, and 5% to cover a bedtime snack if this is required.

Individual Adjustments

All of these doses must be individually adjusted with a written insulin algorithm (see above). Premeal blood glucose targets are 70 to 120 mg/dl for an average teenager or adult. As many as six to eight SMBG determinations a day may be required, with additional nocturnal monitoring, until a pattern emerges and goals are achieved. Many individual patients require larger or smaller proportions of insulin in basal versus bolus mode based on variations in food consumption and activity.

Barriers to Adherence

Even with initial commitment to intensified insulin therapy from the patient and health-care team, problems can arise. Many patients and their families are eager to intensify therapy until they experience the physical, psychological, financial, and practical day-to-day burdens such as continued meal planning, the difficulty of multiple injections or wearing a pump, catheter changes for pump users, more frequent monitoring, and more frequent office visits.

Frustration with persistently variable blood glucose levels despite devoted, even compulsive, efforts ultimately forces some patients into nonadherence. Some patients do well for 3 to 6 months and then slip back into less rigorous patterns of behavior and deteriorating blood glucose control. *Note that when goals of the patient and the health-care team are not congruent, attempts at in-*

tensive insulin therapy are doomed to failure.

Glycosylated hemoglobin determinations not consistent with SMBG reports should raise concern that the patient is not providing honest or accurate data, that psychological problems have been overlooked (e.g., intentionally omitted insulin doses or eating disorders), or, less commonly, that there is a problem in measuring glycosylated hemoglobin.

Hindrances to CSII

Even when a patient's initial commitment persists, the use of pumps may be associated with various problems. These include local abscess formation at catheter sites, pump breakdown and/or malfunction, and forgetting to refill syringes or to change batteries. Undetected air bubbles or occlusions in catheters may obstruct insulin delivery, with resulting hyperglycemia and ketonemia and even diabetic ketoacidosis.

Although some of these difficulties have been partly or completely resolved by the introduction of more flexible infusion sets (which reduce local irritation) and by new buffered insulin preparations (that minimize insulin crystallization and avoid catheter obstruction), the major disadvantage remains the inexorable need for persistent SMBG. This will only be overcome when the need for SMBG is eliminated by implantable glucose sensors and servofeedback with (external or internal) mechanical insulin delivery devices not currently available.

INSULIN ALLERGY

Allergic reactions to insulin are increasingly rare with the widespread use of purified pork and human insulins. However, patients of all ages, particularly those with known atopic diseases, may exhibit local or systemic allergy.

Insulin allergies are more common among users of less pure or more antigenic preparations, e.g., beef or combinations of beef and pork. Some patients may be allergic to the preservatives used in a particular manufacturing process, the protamine in NPH, or the zinc used in high concentrations in the lente series. Isolated cases of allergic reaction to human insulin preparations have been reported.

Some allergic-type reactions may be transient or artifactual. Problems that appear soon after initiation of insulin treatment frequently resolve spontaneously. Burning, itching, and hives at injection sites may result from improper injection technique (intradermal rather than subcutaneous injection or injection of cold insulin) or from localized allergic phenomena.

If symptoms do not resolve and the patient's injection technique is sound, a change from beef and pork insulins to pure pork or human insulin or from one brand or type to another may be in order. True anaphylaxis or severe asthma, although rare, occasionally occurs and should be treated according to well-established protocols (e.g., antihistamines, epinephrine). If changing insulin type does not result in improvement, antihistamines can be prescribed. If atopic phenomena continue or if systemic symptoms occur, consultation with a diabetologist is recommended for alternative approaches, including insulin desensitization.

CONCLUSION

Insulin therapy is the most important aspect of treating the patient with diabetes mellitus.

BIBLIOGRAPHY

Brink SJ: *Pediatric and Adolescent Diabetes Mellitus.* Chicago, IL, Year Book, 1987

Schade DS: *Intensive Insulin Therapy:* Amsterdam, Excerpta Medica, 1983

Monitoring

INTRODUCTION

Monitoring, performed by patients and their health-care providers, is an integral feature of diabetes care. Specifically, results of glucose monitoring are useful in preventing hypoglycemia and adjusting insulin, diet, and exercise so that target blood glucose levels are achieved. Additionally, testing for urine ketones provides an early warning sign of impending ketoacidosis.

PATIENT-PERFORMED MONITORING

Patients can only manage their diabetes effectively and safely if they are able to perform self-monitoring. In certain circumstances (infants or infirm or incapacitated aged patients), monitoring may be performed by family members or health-care providers. Monitoring results must be reviewed periodically and feedback provided by a health-care provider.

Urine Glucose Testing

In the past, the mainstay of diabetes monitoring was urine glucose testing. However, because of its distinct limitations, this method is not ideal as the sole monitoring tool.

Measurement of urinary glucose is an indirect and semiquantitative assessment of the prevailing blood glucose level. Because glycosuria does not occur until the renal threshold is exceeded (usually 160–250 mg/dl), there is a large range of blood glucose levels, from hypoglycemia to frank hyperglycemia, resulting in a negative urine result. Thus, urine testing is not useful in helping the patient discriminate between blood glucose levels in the acceptable range and levels in the hypoglycemic or near-hypoglycemic range. Also, a difference generally exists between the glucose level measured in urine and the level concurrently measured in blood.

Despite its drawbacks, urine testing is easy and inexpensive to perform and may provide general information about blood glucose control. However, the advantages of urine testing are outweighed by the limited information obtained in the insulin-dependent (type I) diabetic patient, necessitating the use of additional monitoring techniques.

Self-Monitoring of Blood Glucose

The most direct method of testing in type I diabetes is self-monitoring of blood glucose (SMBG). This method allows patients to determine their blood glucose levels anywhere (at home, school, work, or while hospitalized), and it allows them to adjust therapy on the basis of accurate and timely results. To perform SMBG, a drop of blood is obtained from a fingertip or earlobe by use of a sharp lancet, usually with the aid of an automatic spring-loaded puncturing device.

The blood is then applied to a chemically impregnated strip, and after a specified time the resulting color change can be quantitated in a meter or read visually by matching it to a reference color chart. Table 7 is a list of commonly used strips, finger-stick devices, and meters for SMBG.

Many commercially available strips and meters have been evaluated and have been shown to be reliable and accurate. With appropriate education, most patients can perform the technique successfully. However, office reassessment of the patient's skills (including the use of a meter if the patient is using one) every 6 to 12 months and the use of quality control techniques at home are essential. Inaccurate measurements can be more dangerous than no measurements at all.

Frequency of SMBG

The frequency and timing of glucose monitoring should be dictated by the particular needs and goals of the patient. At least two tests each day usually provide sufficient information to help adjust insulin and diet. Additional tests before, during, and/or after exercise can help the patient avoid serious hypoglycemia (see **Exercise,** p. 58). For patients who insist on urine testing, even one to two blood tests a day can provide valuable information that will complement urine glucose test results.

Table 7. Products Available for SMBG

FINGER-STICK SUPPLIES

Name and Manufacturer/Distributor	Supplies and Features
Autoclix (Boehringer Mannheim)	Flat design; comes with 3 platforms to vary depth of penetration, 25 lancets
Auto-Lancet (Palco or Orange Medical Instruments)	Comes with 1 adult, 1 juvenile tip (guard), 2 lancets, case. Guard screws on
Autolet (Ames or Ulster Scientific)	Ulster: comes with 20 platforms (10 each of 2 different depths) Ames: comes with 10 platforms (regular depth), 10 lancets, plastic wallet
B-D Autolance (Becton Dickinson)	Flat design; one-piece construction; uses only Microfine lancets specially designed for this unit
Glucolet (Ames)	Comes with 10 Unilet lancets, regular puncture endcaps, super puncture endcaps, instruction insert
Monoject Lancet Device (Sherwood Medical)	Comes with bag of 5 endcaps or box with 10 endcaps; premeasured puncture depth
Penlet (LifeScan)	Clear guard; puncture depth controlled by amount of pressure applied by user
Monoject Lancets (Sherwood Medical) Easy Stik (Diabetes Supplies) TrendsLancets (Orange Medical Instruments)	Can be used alone or in each of the above units except Autolance
Glucosystem Lancets (Ames)	Can be used in either Autolet or Glucolet

TEST STRIPS FOR VISUAL READING

Name and Manufacturer	Instructions for Use
Chemstrip bG (Boehringer Mannheim)	Wipe after 1 min, read; if >240, wait an additional minute, read
Glucostix (Ames)	Blot after 30 s, wait 90 s, read
TrendStrips (Orange Medical Instruments)	Wipe after 1 min, read; if >240, wait an additional minute, read
Visidex II* (Ames)	Blot after 30 s, wait 90 s, read

BLOOD GLUCOSE METERS

Name and Manufacturer	Test Strip Used	Range (mg/dl)
Accu-Chek II (Boehringer Mannheim)	Chemstrip bG	20–500
BetaScan Audio (Orange Medical Instruments)	TrendStrips	0–400
BetaScan B (Orange Medical Instruments)	TrendStrips	0–400
Diascan-S (Home Diagnostics)	Diascan	10–600
Diatron (Diatron Biomedical)	Diatron	11–432
Glucochek SC (EquiMed Medical Products)	Chemstrip bG	10–400
Glucochek SC Audio (EquiMed Medical Products)	Chemstrip bG	10–400
Glucometer II (Ames)	Glucostix	25–399
Glucometer II with memory (Ames)	Glucostix	25–399
Glucometer M (Ames)	Glucostix	25–399
Glucoscan 2000 (LifeScan)	Glucoscan test strips	25–450
Glucoscan 3000 (LifeScan)	Glucoscan test strips	25–450
Tracer (Boehringer Mannheim)	Tracer strips	40–400
TrendsMeter (Orange Medical Instruments)	TrendStrips	0–396

*For visual reading only, other strips listed above can be used with meter or read visually.

Typical testing times include prebreakfast (fasting), prelunch, presupper, and prebedtime. Patients should vary testing times to learn about their blood glucose patterns over the entire day. For patients who are well stabilized on fixed doses of insulin, routine testing (4 times/day) 3 days a week (including 1 weekend day) may be sufficient. Conversely, patients who are ill (see **Education,** p. 24) or whose usual schedule has changed require more frequent monitoring. Box 10 provides typical monitoring schedules depending on intensity of control.

Adjusting Insulin Dose

With SMBG results, patients on a split-mixed regimen can make appropriate insulin adjustments. Occasional unacceptably high or low fasting blood glucose can be treated by adjusting the morning dose of short-acting insulin. If fasting glucose remains in a consistently unacceptable range over a period of days, the evening dose of intermediate-acting insulin should be adjusted.

A late afternoon blood glucose reading can help direct the predinner short-acting insulin and the morning intermediate-acting insulin, which should still be fully effective before dinner. A prebedtime blood glucose reading can help determine the presupper dose and timing of short-acting insulin and the size of the bedtime snack and can occasionally indicate the need for a small additional short-acting insulin supplement. Patients should be encouraged to take notice of persistent glycemic patterns and to correct for them. The dose of long- or intermediate-acting insulin should not be altered because of one odd test result. If blood glucose is *consistently* less than 60 or more than 240 mg/dl (by color estimation) or 300 mg/dl (by meter), or there is persistent ketonuria, the patient should be advised to call the physician.

Pregnant women or other patients who are intensively treated (multiple daily injections or insulin pump regimens) with the goal of achieving near-normal glucose levels will need to perform SMBG more frequently (4–8 times daily) to adjust insulin injections and to avoid hypoglycemia. As with other elements of diabetes management, the prescription for SMBG must be individualized.

Additional Information From SMBG

The value of SMBG is not limited to adjustments in insulin dose. Patients with suspected nocturnal hypoglycemia can check their blood glucose levels at 0300 without being hospitalized (see **Hypoglycemia,** p. 75). SMBG is a

Box 10. Suggested Schedules for SMBG

	Time				
Level of Treatment	Prebreakfast	Prelunch	Predinner	Prebedtime	Other*
Minimal	X - - - - - - - or	- - - - - - - - - X			X
To guide 1 or 2 daily injections of insulin and avoid hypoglycemia. Frequent insulin adjustments not made.					
Average	X		X - - - - or	- - - X	X
To guide 2 daily insulin injections with mixed intermediate and regular insulins. Insulin adjustments made on a more regular basis.					
Intensive	X	X	X	X	X
To guide frequent adjustments of insulin, meals, and exercise when goal is near-normal glycemia. Therapy with at least 3 injections each day or insulin pump.					

*More frequent tests performed on sick days and when ketonuria is present, with changes in exercise or meal pattern, on travel days, or when hypoglycemia is suspected or imminent. Intensively treated patients should perform a 0300-h test on a weekly basis. They may also test 1.5- to 2-h postprandial levels to achieve specified goals. X, time of monitoring.

valuable educational tool to help the patient differentiate between symptoms truly arising from hypoglycemia or hyperglycemia and those from other causes.

Common Causes of Errors

Despite the relative simplicity of SMBG, these methods are not free of errors. The most common problems, independent of specific methodologies, include the use of an inadequate drop of blood on the strip, poor technique in removing blood from the strip, and inaccurate timing. The built-in timers in the latest generation of meters have helped decrease the latter problem. Finally, some patients report their results inaccurately, perhaps to please their physicians with the right results. The use of meters that automatically store glucose results in an electronic memory may simplify the recording and reporting of SMBG. These problems stress the need to provide proper patient education and training in SMBG. At the very least, the package inserts provided with all meters should be mandatory reading for all patients, and the health-care team should test patient familiarity with this information.

Urine Testing for Ketones

Urine testing remains the only practical way to detect ketones (acetone). Even if the patient tests regularly for glucose in blood, the urine *must* be tested for ketones during illness; testing for ketonuria should be a regular feature of sick-day instructions. Additionally, blood glucose levels that are consistently greater than 240 mg/dl by color estimation or 300 mg/dl by meter should prompt the patient to test for ketonuria.

The presence of more than trace amounts of ketones in the urine should prompt patients to call their physicians. Urine ketones are measured with tablets or reagent strips. The latter should be individually wrapped in foil or from a recently opened bottle.

Recording Results

Results of monitoring should be recorded and reviewed by the health-care provider at each office visit. Results can also be phoned or mailed between visits. Health-care professionals must provide appropriate feedback to the patient based on monitoring results.

PHYSICIAN-PERFORMED MONITORING

Because blood glucose levels can fluctuate widely in type I diabetes, sporadic testing in the physician's office is not sufficient as the sole means of monitoring. Intermittent testing does not reliably predict glucose levels at other times or the level of chronic glucose control. Laboratory glucose determinations should be performed occasionally to validate the accuracy of patient-performed monitoring and meter accuracy.

Glycosylated Hemoglobin

The introduction of glycosylated hemoglobin (HbA_1 or HbA_{1c}) assays has revolutionized the ability to follow glucose control over time. When hemoglobin and other proteins are exposed to glucose, the glucose becomes attached to the protein in a slow, nonenzymatic, and concentration-dependent fashion. The concentration of glycosylated hemoglobin best reflects the mean blood glucose concentration over the preceding 6 to 10 weeks.

This measurement is performed on a single tube of blood, and when correctly performed by a reliable lab, the test is unaffected by acute changes in blood glucose; therefore, it can be performed at any time during the day.

Assay Methods

Glycosylated hemoglobin can be assayed with several methods that measure different components of the glycosylated product (e.g., total glycosylated hemoglobin, HbA_{1c}, HbA_1). Depending on the method used, actual test results, including normal ranges, will vary, and results from different laboratories cannot be directly compared. Physicians must determine which assay is being used locally and the nondiabetic range for that assay. Additionally, certain medical conditions, e.g., hemoglobinopathies, polycythemias, and anemias, may affect the results.

Utility

A properly performed glycosylated hemoglobin assay provides the best available index of chronic glucose levels. Other glycosylated protein molecules can be measured for this purpose (e.g., glycosylated albumin), but their role in clinical practice is less well established.

Glycosylated hemoglobin is invaluable in identifying patients who have relatively high, average, or near-normal levels of chronic glucose control. Discrepancies between the glycosylated hemoglobin level and the results of SMBG or urine glucose testing may indicate that the latter are either inaccurately performed or fabricated. A less likely possibility is that the patient has some form of hemoglobinopathy that is interfering with the glycosylated hemoglobin assay: sickle hemoglobin spuriously lowers results, whereas HbF may spuriously elevate glycosylated hemoglobin in some assays.

The measurement of glycosylated hemoglobin allows physician and patient to set objective goals for therapy and to measure the efficacy of changes in therapy. The usual frequency for performing this assay in type I diabetes should be three to four times each year.

CONCLUSION

The appropriate application of self-monitoring techniques (especially SMBG) provides the patient with type I diabetes the opportunity to adjust therapy safely and effectively. The type and frequency of monitoring must be individualized and will be dictated primarily by the patient's life-style and the intensity of insulin therapy. Glycosylated hemoglobin measurements provide an objective index of long-term glucose levels and can be used to determine efficacy of treatment.

BIBLIOGRAPHY

Baynes JW, Bunn HF, Goldstein D, Harris M, Martin DB, Peterson C, Winterhaltar K: National Diabetes Data Group: report of the expert committee on glycosylated hemoglobin. *Diabetes Care* 7:602–608, 1984

Clements RS, Keane NA, Kirk KA, Boshell BR: Comparison of various methods for rapid glucose estimation. *Diabetes Care* 4:392–95, 1981

Goldstein DE, Hoepen MR, Hirsch I, Voluck J: Glucose monitoring: home and office. *Diagnosis* 7:35–46, 1985

Nathan DM, Singer DE, Hurxthal K, Goodson JD: The clinical information value of the glycosylated hemoglobin assay. *N Engl J Med* 310:341–46, 1984

Service FJ, Molnar GD, Taylor WF: Urine glucose analysis during continuous blood glucose monitoring (Abstract). *JAMA* 222:294, 1972

Nutrition

INTRODUCTION

The 1970s and 1980s have brought major revisions in the nutrition management of patients with insulin-dependent (type I) diabetes mellitus. Greater variety in insulin regimens and self-monitoring of blood glucose (SMBG) allows increased flexibility in meal planning. Today's recommended meal plans are higher in complex carbohydrate and lower in protein and fat than their predecessors. Also, there is a somewhat more liberal attitude toward sucrose.

Finally, there has been a convergence of opinions regarding nutrition for the general population and for the patient with diabetes. Current nutrition guidelines of the American Diabetes Association are generally in concert with those for healthy individuals without diabetes, developed by the American Heart Association, the National Research Council, and other national health organizations (Table 8).

Together, these changes mean that nutrition for people with diabetes is increasingly individualized and flexible. More important, they may result in better adherence and improved blood glucose control. The registered dietitian can translate nutrition recommendations into a practical and flexible meal plan.

Table 8. Summary of Nutrient Recommendations and Distribution

NUTRIENT	DISTRIBUTION OF CALORIES (%)	RECOMMENDED DAILY INTAKE
Carbohydrate	55–60	
Fiber		35–40 g/day
Protein	15–20	0.8 g/kg body wt
Fat (total)	<30	
Saturated fat	<10	
Polyunsaturated	≤10	
Monounsaturated	10–15	
Cholesterol		<300 mg/day
Sodium		<3000 mg/day

Data are based on American Diabetes Association: Nutritional recommendations and principles for individuals with diabetes mellitus: 1986 (Position Statement). *Diabetes Care* 10:126–32, 1987

NUTRIENT COMPOSITION: REQUIREMENTS AND RECOMMENDATIONS

Calorie Prescriptions

Calories should be prescribed to achieve and maintain a desirable body weight. Baseline caloric needs take into account height, weight, need for weight loss or gain, and usual activity and/or exercise patterns.

During childhood, adolescence, pregnancy, and lactation, the body requires additional calories. The methods described herein provide guidelines for initially calculating calorie requirements through all phases of the life cycle (Table 9).

Note that for individuals at desired body weight the meal plan for type I diabetes is not intended as a restricted-calorie "diet" but rather as a guideline for *consistency* in food intake to aid in diabetes control. The calorie prescription should also consider weight history and level of metabolic control. To improve metabolic control, it is important to note that fewer calories will be lost through glycosuria and that caloric consumption should be reduced accordingly.

Carbohydrate Needs

The American Diabetes Association's *1986 Nutritional Recommendations* suggest that up to 55 to 60% of total calories can be consumed as carbohydrate, preferably in the form of unrefined high-fiber complex carbohydrate (see Bibliography). If this quantity exceeds previous consumption, intake of complex carbohydrate should be increased gradually, and insulin dose should be adjusted if necessary. Good sources of carbohydrate include whole-grain breads and cereals; pastas, potatoes, beans or peas, and other starches; whole pieces of fruit; and vegetables.

In some individuals whose metabolic control, body weight, and triglyceride levels are satisfactory, sucrose and other refined sugars may occasionally be acceptable. The individual must be educated to adjust insulin and/or to

Table 9. Guidelines for Calculating Calorie Requirements

AGE	CALORIE REQUIREMENTS
0–12 yr	1000 cal for 1st yr + 100 cal/yr over 1
12–15 yr	
Female	1500–2000 cal + 100 cal/yr over 12
Male	2000–2500 cal + 200 cal/yr over 12
15–20 yr	
Female	13–15 cal/lb DBW or 29–33 kcal/kg
Male	15–18 cal/lb DBW or 33–40 kcal/kg
Adults	
Physically active	14–16 cal/lb DBW or 31–35 kcal/kg
Moderately active	12–14 cal/lb DBW or 26–31 kcal/kg
Sedentary	10–12 cal/lb DBW or 22–26 kcal/kg
Sedentary >55 yr, obese and/or inactive	10 cal/lb DBW or 22 kcal/kg
Pregnancy	
1st trimester (2- to 4-lb weight gain)	12–16 cal/lb DBW or 26–35 kcal/kg
2nd and 3rd trimesters (cal may be reduced slightly if obese, early excessive weight gain, sedentary life-style)	13–17 cal/lb DBW or 29–37 kcal/kg
Lactation	15–17 cal/lb DBW or 33–37 kcal/kg

These guidelines aid in *initially* evaluating caloric needs. Calorie requirements and meal plans must periodically be modified to reflect growth and/or weight status and changes in activity and food habits. Optimally, calorie recommendations are based on a nutrition history and assessment that reflects individual's food intake and preferences. DBW, desired body weight.

increase exercise to offset the possible rise in blood glucose from refined carbohydrate and to know the calories, total fat, and types of fat often found in sweets and desserts. These guidelines are provided, not to encourage the use of sweets, but to make meal planning more realistic.

High-Fiber Foods

Some research has found that incorporating high-fiber foods into the meal plan improves carbohydrate metabolism and lowers total cholesterol and low-density lipoprotein levels.

Soluble (as opposed to insoluble) fibers have a major blood glucose–lowering effect. They are found in fruits, legumes, lentils, roots, tubers, oats, and oat bran. Insoluble fibers are found in whole-grain breads and cereals and wheat bran. The *Exchange Lists for Meal Planning* highlights foods with a high fiber content (see Bibliography).

A practical goal is to determine the level of intake (current average 10–30 g/day) and to gradually increase it to perhaps a maximum of 35 to 40 g/day, an amount shown to be beneficial. Individuals who increase fiber intake should be encouraged to increase noncaloric fluid intake as well. Commercial fiber supplements are not recommended. Long-term effects of increased soluble and insoluble fiber intake continue to be investigated.

Higher-fiber foods should be introduced gradually to minimize gastrointestinal problems such as osmotic diarrhea and gas. When increasing fiber intake, patients should be encouraged to pay careful attention to SMBG results, because a high-fiber intake tends to delay and/or reduce peak blood glucose effects from carbohydrate, thereby predisposing to hypoglycemia. Often, insulin dose must be adjusted.

Protein Needs

Although the traditional diabetes meal plan was moderate in protein, the American Diabetes Association's *1986 Nutritional Recommendations* suggests a protein intake of 0.8 $g \cdot kg^{-1}$ body $wt \cdot day^{-1}$* for individuals with diabetes. This is the same as the recom-

*$g \cdot kg^{-1} \cdot min^{-1}$ is often written $g/(kg \cdot min)$ or g/kg/min.

mended daily allowances (RDA) published in 1980. For most adults and children, protein should contribute less than 15 to 20% of total calories. Some research suggests that amounts may be even lower in individuals with nephropathy because reduction in protein may delay the progression of existing renal disease.

Protein sources that are relatively low in total fat, saturated fat, and cholesterol (e.g., fish, poultry, lean red meats, and low-fat cheeses and milk products) are generally better choices than the high-fat protein foods common in the American diet.

Calories From Fat

The current recommendations of the American Diabetes Association suggest that fat contributes less than 30% of total calories. Because this goal may be unrealistically low for Americans, who generally overconsume fat, any reduction should be considered a positive step. Representative high-fat foods include margarine, butter, mayonnaise, salad dressings, gravies, oils, fried foods, and most cheeses.

Polyunsaturated fats should contribute up to 10% of total calories, saturated fats less than 10%, and monounsaturated fats 10 to 15% of total calories. This ratio of saturated to polyunsaturated to monounsaturated fats should remain similar regardless of the percentage of total fat calories contributing to the meal plan. As a practical matter, this goal is best achieved by adhering to the carbohydrate and protein recommendations and restricting fat, cholesterol, and saturated fat intake as suggested by a report from the National Cholesterol Education Program (NCEP) (Table 10).

The American Diabetes Association recommends that individuals with diabetes reduce cholesterol intake to less than 300 mg/day, the same amount specified in the NCEP Step 1 diet of the National Heart, Lung and Blood Institute (see Bibliography). Limiting consumption of eggs (1 medium egg yolk contains ~250 mg cholesterol), cheese, red meats, organ meats, and whole-milk dairy products should decrease cholesterol intake and reduce saturated fat consumption, a major contributor to elevated blood cholesterol levels.

Although some studies suggest that eicosapentaenoic acid (EPA or fish oil) supplements reduce triglycerides and blood cholesterol, current research is too inconclusive to allow a recommendation. Some physicians recommend that fasting cholesterol and triglycerides be monitored at 6- to 12-month intervals.

Table 10. National Cholesterol Education Program: Nutrition Recommendations

NUTRIENT	STEP 1	STEP 2
Total calories from fat	<30%	same
Saturated fat	<10%	<7%
Monounsaturated fat	10–15%	same
Polyunsaturated fat	up to 10%	same
Dietary cholesterol	<300 mg/day	<200 mg/day

Information obtained from National Heart, Lung, and Blood Institute: Report of the National Cholesterol Education Program: expert panel on detection, evaluation, and levels in adults. *Arch Intern Med* 148:36–69, 1988

Sodium Recommendations

A modest sodium intake of less than 3 g/day is generally recommended for diabetic patients. Moderation of sodium intake should be encouraged because of the propensity for high blood pressure and diabetic nephropathy. Individuals susceptible to hypertension, or those in whom it is established, should be especially cautioned against overconsuming sodium. Sodium intake can be minimized by reducing use of table salt, processed and convenience foods, and fast foods. The *Exchange Lists for Meal Planning* highlights foods with a sodium content greater than 400 milligrams per serving.

Vitamins and Minerals

At this time, there is no evidence that vitamin and mineral requirements of individuals with type I diabetes are different from those of other healthy people. If a nutrition assessment reveals a deficiency, individuals should be counseled to increase food intake to meet these needs; only if they are unable to do so should they resort to supplements. However, when caloric intake is less than 1200 cal/day, use of a multivitamin and mineral supplement should be advised. When calcium intake is less than 800 mg/day, supplementation with calcium carbonate up to a total calcium intake of 1000 mg/day is recommended.

MEAL PLANNING FOR TYPE I DIABETIC PATIENTS

As a central feature of diabetes treatment, meal planning should receive prompt attention in the newly diagnosed patient; insulin dosage will be appropriately modified around it. Adjustments in both will be needed periodically.

Meal-Planning Information

Flexible meal-planning schemes, such as an individualized program utilizing the *Exchange Lists for Meal Planning* or a new publication for survival level and lower-level educational needs, *Healthy Food Choices,* can improve adherence (see Bibliography). A preprinted meal plan without nutrition education is clearly not optimal in treating type I patients. Referral to a registered dietitian for nutrition education and the development of an individual meal plan is strongly preferred.

Physicians needing assistance in reaching registered dietitians specialized in diabetes/nutrition management are encouraged to contact the American Diabetes Association or the Diabetes Care and Education Practice Group through the American Dietetic Association. In addition, a professional guide on diabetes nutrition education and counseling and use of the exchange system is available through the American Diabetes Association (see Bibliography). There are other meal-planning systems that can be utilized in diabetes nutrition education. A monograph on meal-planning approaches reviews many of these alternative systems (see Bibliography).

Designing and Implementing the Meal Plan

The physician and dietitian have wide latitude in allocating the amount of calories and carbohydrate to be consumed at each meal and snack. A meal plan should be based on age (young children usually need 3 snacks), growth/weight status, insulin regimen, exercise patterns, and blood glucose results.

Among the *most important considerations* in designing a good meal plan are personal factors, e.g., food habits and schedule. The meal plan should take into account

- food preferences, which are determined by a record of food intake assessed by verbal or written recall;
- the patient's personal time schedule on weekdays and weekends, including school or job, recreation, and social engagements;
- the patient's and, if appropriate, the family's eating habits, including usual time and size of meals and ethnic and cultural preferences; and
- physical activity and its timing.

Although current schedules encourage flexibility, a new meal plan should be adhered to consistently. Day-to-day and meal-to-meal consistency in timing and meal composition (proportion of carbohydrate, protein, and fat) remain the most important factors in achieving optimal blood glucose control. Patients using multiple daily injections or continuous subcutaneous insulin infusion have more liberty in varying quantities at meals and/or changing the times of meals. However, even for them, consistency remains highly desirable.

Regular periodic nutrition consultation to adjust for changes in life-style (e.g., job changes), food preferences, and growth is recommended. In the American Diabetes Association's *Nutritional Recommendations and Principles,* the Task Force on Nutrition recommends that all individuals be seen by a dietitian every 6 months (see Bibliography).

ADDITIONAL NUTRITION CONSIDERATIONS

Sick-Day Management

Individuals with type I diabetes must be educated to manage brief periods when they cannot ingest solid foods. It is imperative for them to understand that *some insulin be continued* and some carbohydrate consumed. Sugar-containing soda or gelatin or apple or cranberry juice can replace the usual carbohydrate in the meal plan. Frequent intermittent intake of small amounts of these foods and other soft beverages helps to avoid hypoglycemia. Individuals should also be taught the importance of ingesting fluids containing sodium and potassium (e.g., vegetable and fruit juices and broths). The usual meal plan should be reintroduced gradually (see **Education,** p. 24 for more on sick-day management).

Growth Years

For infants, children, and adolescents, height and weight data should be plotted on standardized growth grids. Poor diabetes control during the growth years can contribute to failure to attain height potential. During these years, visits with the nutrition counselor should be scheduled every 6 to 12 months to adjust calories and other nutrients and to account for changes in food preferences and habits.

Parents of infants and young children with diabetes may need more frequent nutrition counseling to deal with feeding problems common to young children but that present particular difficulty in type I patients. With most children and adolescents, it is difficult if not impossible to prescribe a meal plan to which the individual can rigidly adhere.

Pregnancy Requirements

The RDA for pregnant women is an additional 300 cal/day over the nonpregnant state [~30–35 kcal/kg (or ~12–16 cal/lb) of desired pregnant body weight; see Table 9 for calorie recommendations during each trimester of pregnancy]. Weight gain should be monitored according to a pregnancy weight-gain chart. Iron and calcium needs are also increased to 75 milligrams of elemental iron and 1200 milligrams of calcium.

During pregnancy, protein allowances are marginally higher than in the nonpregnant state: an additional 30 grams above the adult RDA for protein (0.8 g/kg body wt). However, the meal plans of most women already include enough protein to meet these additional needs. Calories from fat and carbohydrate will stay about the same.

A meal plan of three meals and three to four snacks may be preferable during pregnancy, with one snack eaten at midafternoon and another before bed to prevent nocturnal hypoglycemia and/or ketosis. If there is morning ketosis with normal blood glucose, an increased prebedtime or 0300 h snack should be considered.

Weight loss should not be attempted during pregnancy. Even if the woman begins pregnancy at a higher weight than desired, weight loss should be postponed until after delivery, although weight maintenance is allowable. First-trimester nausea and vomiting must be managed individually.

Lactation Requirements

The RDA for lactation is an additional 500 cal/day, but a slight reduction in calories to produce slow weight loss, if necessary, during lactation is thought to be safe for both mother and infant (see Table 9 for calorie recommendations during lactation). A similar distribution of three meals and three snacks may continue to be desirable during lactation. The calcium and iron requirements are similar to those suggested during pregnancy. Women who are breast-feeding are often advised to continue taking a prenatal vitamin and/or mineral supplement.

Obesity Management

With the initiation of insulin therapy, weight lost before diagnosis is most often regained, and excessive weight gain may continue for several reasons, e.g., overinsulinization, overtreatment of insulin reactions, efforts to avoid insulin reactions with the use of extra food, failure to decrease calorie intake to compensate for decreased urinary calorie loss, and general emphasis on food intake.

Parents and diabetic individuals should be advised about the consequences of obesity on general health. Individuals with diabetes mellitus who are attempting to lose weight should avoid any fad diets that promote inappropriate food combinations and rapid weight loss, because dehydration, fluid and electrolyte imbalances, and starvation ketosis may result. Weight-loss programs for individuals with type I diabetes must include advice about insulin dose adjustment, careful monitoring of diabetes control, and realistic weight-loss goals. The safety of the weight-loss program must be paramount.

Eating Disorders

An increasing number of children, adolescents, and adults in the general population appear to be affected with anorexia nervosa, bulimia, or a combination of the two. Type I diabetes mellitus complicated by an eating disorder is very difficult to manage because of erratic eating patterns and purging behaviors such as vomiting, laxative abuse, or excessive exercise.

A purging behavior unique to type I diabetes is self-induced glycosuria, achieved by overeating with underinsulinization. If these destructive behaviors persist despite the expertise of the managing health-care provider, referral to appropriate medical, psychological, and nutrition counselors is strongly urged.

Alternative Sweeteners

Use of alternative sweeteners, both caloric and noncaloric, is acceptable for individuals with type I diabetes. Moderate use of alternative sweeteners should be advised within established safe levels to prevent chronic use by type I diabetic patients. Individuals may be encouraged to use various alternative sweeteners to decrease intake of any one product (see Bibliography).

Saccharin is noncaloric, and aspartame is virtually noncaloric, although for tabletop use, both are packaged with dextrose and contain about 4 calories per packet. Aspartame is marketed as NutraSweet for incorporation into reduced-calorie and/or sugar-free products. As a tabletop sweetener, it is known as Equal. Saccharin is found in Sweet'N Low and Sugar Twin.

Sorbitol and fructose constitute a category referred to as caloric sweeteners. They are often incorporated into foods (cake mixes, candy bars, and cookies) that are technically sugar free but may be calorically equivalent to the non–sugar-free products they mimic and may elevate blood glucose. Individuals should be warned against using these products freely. Sorbitol may also have a laxative effect, causing osmotic diarrhea and/or abdominal cramping.

Use of Alcohol

With the exception of individuals whose blood glucose is out of control, those attempting weight loss, those with elevated blood triglycerides, and pregnant women, most adults with type I diabetes may drink alcohol in moderation. Two ounces of alcohol one to two times a week appears to be prudent.

In addition to the precautions regarding alcohol use that apply to the general public, people with type I diabetes risk

Table 11. Alcohol and Nutrient Content of Common Alcoholic Beverages

ITEM	AVERAGE SERVING (oz)	ALCOHOL (g/serving)	CHO (g/serving)	CALORIES per serving	EXCHANGE VALUES
Beer (regular)	12	13.0	13.7	151	2 fats and 1 starch
Beer (low cal)	12	10.1	5.1	97	2 fats
Table wine					
Red	4	11.6	0.2	83	2 fats
White	4	11.6	0.4	80	2 fats
Distilled spirits (86 proof, i.e., gin, whiskey, vodka, scotch, rum)	1.5	15.3		107	2 fats

Information obtained from McDonald J: Alcohol and diabetes. *Diabetes Care* 3:629–37, 1980

alcohol-induced hypoglycemia when meals are skipped or during fasting. Therefore, it is no longer recommended that the calories be reduced to balance calories derived from alcohol. However, if the patient is on a weight-loss regimen, calories from alcohol must be considered, and intake should be minimal.

Two ounces of alcohol may be consumed in addition to the regular meal plan, but patients should be advised to consume food either at the time of alcohol intake or before bed if alcohol is consumed later in the evening. Also, excessive alcohol may impair recognition of hypoglycemia and ability to counterregulate. Patients should avoid sweetened alcoholic mixed drinks, liqueurs, and after-dinner alcoholic drinks because of their increased sugar content (Table 11).

Glycemic Indexing of Foods

Carbohydrate foods that were formerly assumed to cause similar elevations of blood glucose are now known to have differing glycemic effects. The glycemic index is a method to measure the glycemic effect of foods. However, so many variables affect the rate at which blood glucose rises that the index is of limited usefulness and is not generally applicable or teachable.

Motivated individuals who closely monitor the effects of various foods on their blood glucose may find glycemic indexing helpful. They should seek the counsel of a dietitian able to assist in this procedure.

Box 11. Continuing Nutrition Counseling on Diabetes

- Periodic meal plan revisions based on life-style changes and needs
- Reinforcement of basic principles of meal planning
- Food recommendations for exercise
- Sick-day management
- Weight-control strategies
- Restaurant, fast food, and ethnic dining skills
- Appropriate use of alcohol
- Increasing fiber intake
- Use of alternative sweeteners
- Food preparation methods (low-fat, low-cholesterol cooking and alternative sweeteners in baking)
- Incorporating convenience foods and favorite recipes
- Recommendations for resources, e.g., magazines, cookbooks, books

Ongoing nutrition education is optimally provided by a dietitian familiar with diabetes management.

NUTRITION EDUCATION

At diagnosis, nutrition counseling should emphasize "survival skills," the basic information needed during the first few weeks of diabetes. Health-care professionals working with newly diagnosed diabetic patients should be prepared to provide survival level nutrition guidelines. These include basic meal planning and eating principles, managing unanticipated exercise, and recognizing and treating hypoglycemia. *Healthy Food Choices* is useful in teaching initial meal planning skills (see Bibliography). As soon as possible, the patient and/or family should see a registered dietitian for more in-depth and ongoing nutrition counseling (Box 11). A wide variety of teaching tools in various types of media for many educational levels has been developed on diabetes meal planning.

Because of the pivotal role of nutrition in maintaining the health of the patient with diabetes, third-party reimbursement for a registered dietitian's services is becoming increasingly available, especially when initiated by a physician referral.

CONCLUSION

Along with insulin, nutrition is one of the major pillars in the treatment of diabetes mellitus. Knowledge of meal planning, regularity of food intake, flexibility in food choices, and adherence within recommended caloric levels facilitates metabolic control and constitutes prescriptions for healthy living rather than a special diet that connotes restriction.

BIBLIOGRAPHY

American Diabetes Association: Nutritional recommendations and principles for individuals with diabetes mellitus: 1986 (Position Statement). *Diabetes Care* 10:126, 1987

American Diabetes Association: Report of the American Diabetes Association's Task Force on Nutrition. *Diabetes Care* 11: 127–211, 1988

American Diabetes Association and American Dietetic Association: *Exchange Lists for Meal Planning.* Alexandria, VA, Am. Diabetes Assoc., and Chicago, IL, Am. Dietetic Assoc., 1986

American Diabetes Association and American Dietetic Association: *Healthy Food Choices.* Alexandria, VA, Am. Diabetes Assoc., and Chicago, IL, Am. Dietetic Assoc., 1986

American Diabetes Association and American Dietetic Association: *Family Cookbook.* Vols. I and II, New York, Prentice Hall, 1987

American Diabetes Association and American Dietetic Association: *Family Cookbook.* Vol. III, New York, Prentice Hall, 1987

American Diabetes Association and American Dietetic Association: *Nutritional Guide for Professionals: Diabetes Education and Meal Planning.* Alexandria, VA, Am. Diabetes Assoc., and Chicago, IL, Am. Dietetic Assoc., 1988

American Dietetic Association: *Diabetes Nutrition Information Series.* Chicago, IL, Am. Dietetic Assoc., 1986

American Dietetic Association: *Ethnic and Regional Food Practices.* Chicago, IL, Am. Dietetic Assoc. In press

Crapo P: Use of noncaloric sweeteners (Position Statement). *Diabetes Care* 10:526, 1987

Holler H, Green J: *Meal Planning Approaches in the Nutritional Management of the Person With Diabetes Mellitus.* Chicago, IL, Am. Dietetic Assoc., 1987

Powers M: *Handbook of Diabetes and Nutritional Management.* Rockville, MD, Aspen, 1987

Wedman B: *American Diabetes Association Holiday Cookbook.* New York, Prentice Hall, 1986

Exercise

INTRODUCTION

In addition to insulin and the meal plan, exercise plays a key role in diabetes treatment; a *specific* exercise program should be part of the treatment plan for *all* patients with insulin-dependent (type I) diabetes mellitus. Increased activity may improve glycemic control, help control weight, bring about a healthier mental outlook, and reduce cardiovascular risk factors.

Given appropriate guidelines, people with diabetes can exercise safely. Children and adolescents can participate fully in gym classes, team sports, and other activities. Most adults should exercise more regularly and more vigorously. Even incapacitated people can be taught how to exercise safely and should be encouraged to do so.

The exercise plan will vary for each patient depending on interest, age, general health, and level of physical fitness. For some, mild exercise may be prescribed (e.g., walking 0.50–1.0 mile at a comfortable pace with heart rate <60% of maximum capacity for age). Other patients may benefit most from moderate exercise (e.g., walking 1–1.5 miles at a brisk pace, with heart rate <70% of maximum capacity for age). For patients who are reasonably fit, strenuous exercise of sufficient duration and intensity to promote a training or endurance effect can be recommended (e.g., jogging 2–3 miles with heart rate 70–90% of maximum capacity for age).

GLYCEMIC RESPONSE TO EXERCISE

Exercise requires rapid mobilization and redistribution of metabolic fuels to ensure an adequate energy supply for muscle contraction. In nondiabetic people, this complex process is coordinated via neural and hormonal responses that increase production of glucose and free fatty acids (FFA) and facilitate uptake and utilization of glucose by muscle (Box 12).

In nondiabetic people, insulin levels fall while counterregulatory hormones rise, so increased glucose utilization of exercising muscle is matched *precisely* by increased glucose production from liver. In patients with type I diabetes, the glycemic response to exercise varies depending on overall diabetes control, plasma glucose levels at the start of exercise, intensity and duration of the exercise, and previous conditioning.

The important variable is the level of plasma insulin attained during and after exercise. Exercise increases blood flow and therefore the rate of insulin absorption from subcutaneous sites. Thus, although insulin levels in nondiabetic people will fall, in diabetic patients they may rise. Excessive insulin levels can potentiate hypoglycemia because of insulin-enhanced muscle glucose uptake and inhibition of the rate of hepatic glucose production. The magnitude of the discrepancy between the rate of glucose use versus the rate of glucose production determines the timing and severity of hypoglycemia. By contrast, in the already poorly controlled (underinsulinized) patient, the insulin levels are too low, so that with the rise in counterregulatory hormones during exercise, production of glucose and FFA continue, whereas uptake is minimal, resulting in large increases in plasma glucose and ketone levels.

POTENTIAL BENEFITS OF EXERCISE

Clear-cut cardiovascular benefits accrue to patients who participate in endurance training programs. However, many other advantages, e.g., weight control and improved sense of well-being, can be achieved with even modest exercise programs that do not reach the intensity of endurance training.

Physical training *reduces risk factors for cardiovascular disease.* Exercise is associated with a reduction in circulating levels of very-low-density lipoprotein (VLDL) and low-density lipoprotein (LDL) cholesterol and triglycerides and with an increase in high-density lipoprotein (HDL) cholesterol, which is thought to protect against cardiovascular disease. In addition, exercise reduces blood pressure and increases cardiac work capacity.

When combined with a well-struc-

Box 12. Response to Exercise: The Role of Insulin

In nondiabetic people, insulin plays a key role in integrating production and use of fuels for exercising muscle. In insulin-treated diabetic people, response to exercise will vary depending on the insulin level, which may rise and/or fall during exercise.

Response in Nondiabetic People

+UTILIZATION of glucose	+PRODUCTION of glucose, free fatty acids
■ Uptake into exercising muscle	■ Counterregulatory hormones stimulate output
■ Insulin: moderate decrease, still adequate for uptake	■ Insulin: moderate decrease promotes output

Result: precise *integration* of fuel utilization and production

Response in Type I People

INSULIN EXCESS

Occurs because increased blood flow during exercise accelerates rate of absorption from subcutaneous sites

++UTILIZATION of glucose	−PRODUCTION of glucose, free fatty acids
■ Uptake into exercising muscle	■ Counterregulatory hormones stimulate output
■ Insulin excess facilitates uptake	■ Insulin excess restrains output

Result: greater utilization and restrained production result in *hypoglycemia.* This may occur *during* or *after* exercise

INSULIN LACK

Occurs in poorly controlled (underinsulinized) patients

−UTILIZATION of glucose	++PRODUCTION of glucose, FFA
■ Uptake into exercising muscle	■ Counterregulatory hormones stimulate output
■ Insulin lack blocks uptake	■ Insulin lack greatly promotes output

Result: greater production and diminished utilization result in *hyperglycemia* and *ketonemia,* which may progress to ketoacidosis

+, Increased; ++, greatly increased; −, decreased or inadequate.

tured meal plan, regular exercise can make *weight loss or weight maintenance* much easier. This may be of special benefit to patients controlled at intensive levels.

Physical activity *improves glycemic control* by increasing insulin sensitivity. Studies indicate that glycosylated hemoglobin levels significantly improve with exercise if the exercise is carefully integrated into a total-care program that includes meal-plan adherence and frequent self-monitoring of blood glucose (SMBG).

Regular physical activity can ease the psychological stress often associated with a busy modern-day life-style. People who engage in regular exercise experience an *improved sense of well-being*; for them, exercise becomes an important and pleasurable part of their daily routine.

POTENTIAL RISKS OF EXERCISE

As with other medical therapies, *exercise has risks as well as benefits.*

Box 13. Precautions for Patients With Medical Complications

- Insensitive feet or peripheral vascular insufficiency—avoid running; choose walking, cycling, swimming
- Active proliferative retinopathy—avoid exercises associated with increased intra-abdominal pressure, Valsalva-like maneuvers, or acceleration-deceleration trauma to the head
- Hypertension—avoid heavy lifting and Valsalva-like maneuvers; choose exercises that involve the lower- rather than primarily upper-extremity muscle groups

Effect on Glycemic Control

Because prolonged and strenuous exercise can potentiate the effects of insulin, hypoglycemia during or after exercise is a definite risk for the individual with type I diabetes. It is a particular risk for patients who exercise sporadically while continuing to take their usual insulin dose.

Individual response patterns differ markedly. Some people regularly develop hypoglycemia during moderate exercise if no supplemental food is taken immediately before the activity, whereas others become hypoglycemic only many hours after the exercise. Because all patients with type I diabetes have some periods of relative insulin excess, it may be necessary to time the exercise so that it does not coincide with periods of peak insulin absorption. Conversely, if diabetes is controlled at a minimal level or blood glucose is high before beginning activity, exercise may worsen metabolic control to the point of diabetic ketoacidosis.

Box 14. Guidelines for Safe Exercise

Tell all patients to

- carry an identification card and wear a bracelet at all times that identifies them as having diabetes;
- be alert for signs of hypoglycemia during and for several hours after exercise;
- have immediate access to a source of readily absorbable carbohydrate (such as glucose tablets) to treat hypoglycemia;
- take sufficient fluids before, after, and if necessary, during exercise to prevent dehydration; and
- measure blood glucose. Take appropriate action if <80 or >240 mg/dl by color estimation and >300 mg/dl with a meter.

Other Risk Factors

Because patients with diabetes have an increased incidence of cardiovascular disease, there is the risk that exercise will precipitate arrhythmia, myocardial ischemia, or infarction. Risks related to underlying retinopathy and neuropathy and the inability to prevent hypoglycemia must be carefully considered. As in nondiabetic individuals, exercise can also aggravate preexisting joint disease or cause musculoskeletal injuries.

REDUCING EXERCISE RISKS

Potential hazards can be prevented or reduced if the exercise program is preceded by a medical evaluation, well supervised, and planned to progress gradually from low to more strenuous levels of exertion.

Preexercise Medical Evaluation

The preexercise medical evaluation should be performed regardless of the patient's age and should include

- assessment of glycemic control, including a glycosylated hemoglobin determination;
- cardiovascular examination, including an ECG at rest and with exercise if the patient is more than 30 years old and/or has had diabetes for more than 15 years;
- neurologic and musculoskeletal examinations, including an examination of the feet; and
- ophthalmologic examination (by an ophthalmologist if retinopathy is present).

Exercise should be prescribed with caution in patients with minimally controlled blood glucose; cardiovascular disease, neuropathy, or proliferative retinopathy; and/or inability to prevent hypoglycemia (hypoglycemic unawareness). These patients will need to choose types of exercise judiciously (Box 13). They should avoid intense exercise, but moderate exercise is acceptable and even encouraged if the patient desires.

Patients with known cardiovascular complications should have an exercise program developed through a cardiac rehabilitation program. Special precautions are also required in patients taking drugs that could precipitate hypoglycemia (e.g., beta-adrenergic–blocking agents) or in people with other medical conditions such as hyperthyroidism or hypertension.

Instructions to Patients

All exercising patients should be given specific instructions regarding choice of exercise, glycemic control during exercise, and monitoring intensity of exercise and should take appropriate safety measures (Box 14). At each clinic visit the physician should review the risks of hypoglycemia and the dangers of exercise if diabetes is minimally controlled.

THE EXERCISE PRESCRIPTION

Exercise should be prescribed for the patient in much the same way as the meal plan and insulin. The key to success is *individualization*. The exercise program must be designed with the patient's input, taking into account age, life-style, stage of physical conditioning, and motivation. Similarly, the duration, frequency, and intensity of exercise, as well as the type chosen, must be mutually determined. Table 12 outlines exercise prescriptions based on a range of initial fitness levels.

An endurance training program is desirable for almost everyone with diabetes. However, some patients will be physically unable or otherwise unwilling to undertake such a program; for these patients, a more modest program of *regular* exercise should be arranged. Patients reluctant to exercise regularly should be advised that even brief, infrequent exercise, properly performed, is better than none at all and that increases in normal daily activities (e.g., walking and climbing stairs) are useful adjuncts to the diabetes program.

Whenever possible, an "exercise contract" should be arranged with the patient. The agreed-on plan should be carefully documented and the patient's adherence to the program reviewed regularly and revised as needed. It is not enough just to tell patients that exercise is important and that they should do it regularly; few patients (or physicians) will respond positively to unstructured recommendations.

Endurance Training

Patients who are interested and physically able should be encouraged to participate in endurance training. Endurance training stimulates cardiovascular fitness by using a large portion of the skeletal muscle mass for at least 15 to 30 minutes three times per week at 60 to 90% of maximum heart-rate capacity (Table 13). Highly trained athletes may reach levels of 90% or more, although levels above 80% of maximum do not appear to promote further endurance. Thus, a person who rides a sta-

Table 12. Exercise Prescriptions

FITNESS LEVEL	FREQUENCY (min)	DURATION (sessions/wk)	INTENSITY (min/session)	PERCENT OF MAXIMUM HEART RATE
Very low	40–80	4–6	10–20	60
Low	90–120	4–6	15–30	60–70
Moderate	120–180	3–5	30–45	70–80
High	180–300	3–5	30–60	70–80
Athlete	300–840	5–7	60–120	70–90

Adapted from Vignati LV, Cunningham LN: Exercise and diabetes. In *Joslin's Diabetes Mellitus*. Marble A, White P, Bradley RF, Krall LP, Eds. Philadelphia, PA, Lea & Febiger, 1985, chapt. 22, p. 460

tionary bicycle for 30 minutes but raises the heart rate to only 40% of maximum predicted for age has not done much to improve cardiovascular fitness. This person would need to pedal faster, longer, and/or against greater resistance until heart rate and duration goals are achieved.

If the clinician does not feel knowledgeable enough to personally prescribe and supervise a strenuous exercise program, the patient should be referred to one of the many programs available through physical education departments of colleges, hospitals (particularly cardiac rehabilitation programs), and health and fitness clubs.

PREPARING FOR EXERCISE: ADJUSTING FOOD AND INSULIN

The meal plan and insulin dosage should be adjusted according to the patient's own response to physical activity. Because there is greater variability in responses, it is helpful for patients to monitor blood glucose before, during, and after exercise to learn their own response pattern. Generally, blood glucose values under 80 mg/dl indicate the need for a snack; those over 240 mg/dl by color estimation and over 300 mg/dl with a meter indicate the need to adjust insulin or delay exercise.

Adjusting Calorie Intake

Moderate exercise of less than 30 to 45 minutes rarely requires any insulin adjustment, but often a small snack is needed just before the exercise, especially if blood glucose is less than 80 mg/dl. Longer periods of exercise almost always require snacks every 30 to 60 minutes.

Experts differ in their recommendations for the type of food to be given. A serving of approximately 15 to 20 grams of a rapidly absorbed carbohydrate is quite effective in preventing hypoglycemia but may raise the blood glucose level excessively. For this reason, some nutrition experts favor snacks containing a mixture of complex carbohydrate and protein (try approximately ½ meat or milk exchange and ½ bread exchange, which is equivalent to 60–90 cal).

Both approaches appear to work well. The actual snack size required to prevent hypoglycemia must be determined on an individual basis and will vary depending on the duration and intensity of the activity. Patients who typically experience hypoglycemia only several hours after the exercise should take a snack after the exercise. For the patient who exercises in the evening, it is particularly important to monitor for nocturnal hypoglycemia and adjust the evening snack as appropriate.

Table 13. Exercise Heart Rate by Age

AGE (yr)	PREDICTED MAXIMAL HEART RATE	PERCENT OF MAXIMAL HEART RATE						
		90	85	80	75	70	65	60
15	193	174	164	154	145	135	125	116
20	191	172	162	153	143	134	124	115
25	189	170	161	151	142	133	123	113
30	186	167	158	149	140	130	121	111
35	184	166	156	147	138	129	120	110
40	182	164	155	146	137	127	118	109
45	180	162	153	144	135	126	117	108
50	178	160	151	142	134	125	116	107
55	175	158	149	140	131	123	114	105
60	173	156	147	138	130	121	112	104
65	171	154	145	137	128	120	111	103

Adapted from Vignati LV, Cunningham LN: Exercise and diabetes. In *Joslin's Diabetes Mellitus.* Marble A, White P, Bradley RF, Krall LP, Eds. Philadelphia, PA, Lea & Febiger, 1985, chapt. 22, p. 459

Adjusting Insulin

Sometimes it is necessary to adjust the insulin dosage to prevent hypoglycemia. This occurs most often with strenuous activity of greater than 45 to 60 minutes duration. The specific adjustment will depend on the patient's insulin dose regimen. For most patients, a small decrease (~20%) in the short-acting insulin component of the injection before exercise is sufficient to prevent hypoglycemia. However, this approach may lead to late hyperglycemia, necessitating a supplemental injection of short-acting insulin before the main meal after the exercise. If possible, patients should avoid injecting insulin in the extremity that will be predominantly used for the exercise.

For very prolonged vigorous exercise, such as backpacking or long-distance cycling, a large decrease in the total daily insulin dosage (by as much as ⅓ to ½) may be necessary to prevent repeated hypoglycemic episodes. In this case, both short- and longer-acting insulin components should be decreased proportionally.

In contrast to these acute reductions in insulin dosage, individuals participating in long-term fitness programs often find that the total daily dosage of insulin will decrease by as much as 15 to 20%.

MONITORING INTENSITY OF EXERCISE

Regular participation in moderate or strenuous exercise is safer and can be quantitated more easily if patients know how to monitor exercise intensity by assessing heart rate and sense of fatigue. Patients can be taught how to monitor heart rate by palpating the carotid or radial pulse or by simply placing the hand on the left anterior chest wall.

The patient should take a 10-second count during the exercise or within 5 seconds of stopping and multiply the result by 6 to determine heart rate per minute. Patients should be alerted to stop exercising immediately if they experience extreme discomfort or pain, severe shortness of breath, lightheadedness, or nausea.

Patients starting from a low level of fitness should also check their heart rate 5 and 10 minutes after the exercise session. It should be less than 120 and 100 beats per minute, respectively. Shortness of breath should not be present after 5 to 7 minutes of rest.

Each session of moderate or strenuous exercise should include a warm-up and a cool-down period. Five to ten minutes of stretching and flexibility exercises should be followed by more vigorous exercises, and the session should be concluded with 10 to 20 minutes of less strenuous exercises and stretching. For the person who is poorly conditioned at the start, initial goals should always be very modest, starting with short (5–10 min) but frequent (5–7 days/wk) sessions.

CONCLUSION

Long called a cornerstone of diabetes treatment, exercise is underestimated as a therapeutic modality; its hazards are too often perceived to outweigh its benefits. However, working with guidelines such as those supplied herein, physicians can frame a safe program of regular exercise that promotes the health and well-being of their type I patients.

BIBLIOGRAPHY

Astrand PO: Aerobic work capacity in men and women with special reference to age. *Acta Physiol Scand Suppl* 169:1, 1960

Cooper KH: *The New Aerobics.* New York, Evans, 1981

Vignati L, Cunningham LN: Exercise and Diabetes. In *Joslin's Diabetes Mellitus.* Marble A, White P, Bradley RF, Krall LP, Eds. Philadelphia, PA, Lea & Febiger, 1985, chapt. 22, p. 453–64

Zinman B, Vranic M: Diabetes and exercise. *Med Clin N Am* 69:145–56, 1985

Special Problems

Highlights
Special Problems

DIABETIC KETOACIDOSIS

Diabetic ketoacidosis (DKA) is a life-threatening but reversible complication characterized by severe disturbances in protein, fat, and carbohydrate regulation.

DKA is always due to insulin deficiency, either absolute (e.g., a previously undiagnosed patient or omitted insulin) or relative (e.g., too little insulin injected or antagonism by stress hormones).

Any major stress may precipitate DKA in a patient with diabetes who lacks sufficient circulating insulin.

The clinical signs and symptoms of DKA are listed in Box 15, page 64. They usually include polyuria, polydipsia, hyperventilation, dehydration, the fruity odor of ketones, and disturbances in the conscious state from drowsiness to frank coma.

The initial goal of therapy should be to correct life-threatening abnormalities, i.e.,

- dehydration,
- insulin deficiency, or
- potassium deficiency.

Frequent reexamination of laboratory indices is imperative: at minimum, every hour during the first 4 hours and at least every 4 hours thereafter.

Routine bicarbonate administration is not recommended. Conservative potassium phosphate administration is recommended for all patients. Some patients may require more aggressive therapy.

The cause of DKA must be aggressively pursued. Potential complications of therapy and how to avoid them are outlined on page 68.

DKA can often be prevented, given appropriate patient education and prompt physician attention.

HYPOGLYCEMIA

Hypoglycemia is a common side effect of insulin therapy. Mild hypoglycemic reactions usually consist of adrenergic symptoms, e.g., tremors, palpitations, sweating, and excessive hunger. Moderate and severe reactions include neuroglycopenic and adrenergic symptoms.

Mild hypoglycemic reactions are only a nuisance. **Moderate and severe insulin reactions may severely harm health and morale and should be avoided.**

Certain circumstances favor development of prolonged, incapacitating, and occasionally life-threatening hypoglycemia, i.e.,

- hypoglycemic unawareness,
- delayed treatment, or
- failure to notice symptoms because attention is elsewhere or during sleep.

The factors precipitating an episode of hypoglycemia can often be identified, allowing prevention of future reactions in similar circumstances (p. 72).

Self-monitoring of blood glucose (SMBG) should be used to full advantage for detection and treatment of hypoglycemia. Changes in insulin injection, eating, or exercise schedules and travel call for increased frequency of monitoring.

Guidelines for treatment of mild (p. 73), moderate (p. 74), and severe (p. 74) reactions should be clearly understood by patient, family, and school and business associates.

Hypoglycemia with rebound hyperglycemia should be recognized and appropriately treated (p. 74); otherwise, a cycle of overinsulinization may result.

PREGNANCY

Women with type I diabetes who receive optimal care by an experienced health-care team can expect a pregnancy outcome similar to that of women who do not have diabetes.

Excellent glycemic control during pregnancy has been shown to bring

unequivocally beneficial results to both mother and fetus.

Poor perinatal outcome is associated with long-standing diabetes, poor glycemic control, and vasculopathy.

Patients should be as near to normoglycemia as possible at the time of conception and throughout the first trimester to decrease incidence of congenital malformations.

Self-monitoring of blood glucose (SMBG) is mandatory during pregnancy.

Most women with type I diabetes may be managed as outpatients throughout gestation.

Tests to assess fetal growth and well-being should be conducted at appropriate times (p. 81). **Timing of delivery and management during labor and delivery** are covered on page 82. Postpartum care is covered on page 83. **Family planning and contraception** must be reviewed with the patient during the postpartum period (p. 83).

SURGERY

Given appropriate preparation and management, patients with type I diabetes are subject to little more than normal risk during surgery.

Whenever possible, the patient should be in the best possible general health and glycemic control before a surgical procedure.

The objectives of glycemic management before, during, and after an operation are to prevent hypoglycemia and excessive hyperglycemia and ketoacidosis.

Because hypoglycemia is particularly dangerous, plasma glucose is generally kept between approximately 150 and 250 mg/dl during and after the operation.

Intravenous insulin delivery is preferred during surgery.

In patients with diabetic ketoacidosis (DKA) who need emergency surgery, efforts should be made to delay surgery until DKA is treated.

Guidelines for surgery:

- major elective surgery, page 84
- major emergency surgery, page 84
- surgery with local anesthesia, page 85

Diabetic Ketoacidosis

INTRODUCTION

Diabetic ketoacidosis (DKA) is a life-threatening but reversible complication characterized by severe disturbances in protein, fat, and carbohydrate regulation that results from insulin deficiency. DKA is considered to be a medical emergency requiring treatment in a medical intensive care unit or equivalent setting.

In DKA, the arterial pH is less than 7.2, plasma bicarbonate is less than or equal to 15 meq/L, blood glucose is generally greater than 250 mg/dl, and ketones are in the blood and urine. DKA is always due to insulin deficiency, either absolute or relative. It is absolute as the initial condition in a previously undiagnosed patient whose metabolic condition progresses to DKA or because a patient omitted a scheduled insulin injection. It is relative when too little insulin is administered or there is insufficient biologic activity of the insulin at the tissues because of the influence of counterregulatory hormones.

The counterregulatory or stress hormones comprise glucagon, catecholamines, cortisol, and growth hormone and are markedly elevated in DKA. Acting in concert, they antagonize the biologic effects of insulin and augment the metabolic derangements characteristic of DKA by promoting

- hyperglycemia secondary to increased glucose production and decreased utilization,
- osmotic diuresis and dehydration secondary to hyperglycemia,
- hyperlipemia secondary to increased lipolysis,
- acidosis secondary to increased production and decreased utilization of acetoacetic acid and 3-beta-hydroxybutyric acid derived from fatty acids, especially with dehydration and diminished renal blood flow, and
- an increased anion gap secondary to elevated ketoacids and lactate.

PRESENTATION OF DKA

The clinical diagnosis of DKA is usually apparent in a patient known to have insulin-dependent (type I) diabetes. However, DKA may not be readily considered at first in an elderly, comatose patient with non-insulin-dependent (type II) diabetes or in a child with new-onset diabetes whose rapid breathing is perceived as pneumonia. The diagnosis may also be confused with alcoholic ketoacidosis or starvation ketosis, because both conditions induce ketonemia and acidosis. A blood glucose concentration less than 250 mg/dl usually excludes DKA unless the patient has been partially treated by additional insulin and fluids before presentation.

Clinical Signs and Symptoms

The clinical signs and symptoms of DKA usually include polyuria, polydipsia, hyperventilation, and dehydration (Box 15). The fruity odor of ketones will be apparent, and disturbances in conscious state vary from drowsiness to frank coma. Abdominal pain in association with an elevated white blood cell count and serum amylase may occur, particularly in young people, but it usually resolves with therapy. If severe abdominal pain persists, a surgical consultation should be obtained, because an acute condition such as appendicitis, bowel perforation, or infarction may exist.

Precipitating Factors

Any major stress may precipitate DKA in a diabetic patient who lacks sufficient circulating insulin. Infections such as pneumonia, meningitis, gastroenteritis, and influenza are some of the many heterogeneous causes as are trauma, myocardial infarction, and stroke. In most patients, it is possible to identify a specific precipitating cause. Among the most common are deliberate or inadvertent omission of insulin and mismanagement of sick days (withholding insulin from a patient who is vomiting and unable to eat, mistakenly believing it may provoke hypoglycemia) (Box 16).

ACUTE PATIENT CARE

The initial goal of therapy should be to correct *life-threatening abnormalities, i.e., dehydration, insulin deficiency, and*

Box 15. Common Presenting Symptoms and Signs in Diabetic Ketoacidosis

SYMPTOMS	SIGNS
Nausea and vomiting	Tachycardia
Thirst and polyuria	Hypotension
Weakness and/or anorexia	Dehydration
Abdominal pain	Warm dry skin
Visual disturbances	Hyperventilation
Somnolence	Impaired consciousness and/or coma
	Weight loss

potassium deficiency. This must be done with great care. Fully correcting all biochemical abnormalities may take as long as 1 week after the patient is eating solid foods.

Correct treatment of DKA is a feasible goal for all physicians. Frequent reexamination of laboratory indices is imperative to prevent serious electrolyte imbalance and fluid overload. During the first 12 hours of therapy, the condition should be reevaluated *at least* hourly in the first 4 hours and at least every 4 hours thereafter. Particular attention should be paid to plasma potassium concentration. A flow sheet tabulating successive changes in the patient's condition must be maintained for all patients (Box 17). If the patient's clinical condition deteriorates after initial therapy has begun or if a metabolic complication occurs, consultation with an appropriate specialist is strongly recommended.

The degree of hyperglycemia, acidosis, dehydration, and conscious state is variable and depends partly on whether gluconeogenesis, lipolysis, or ketogenesis is the predominating metabolic abnormality. Other factors include the nutritional state of the patient, duration of DKA, concurrent drug therapy, degree of insulin deficiency, and the individual's inherent metabolism (see Bibliography). For a recommended treatment schedule, see Boxes 18–20. Individual patients may require different replacement schedules depending on clinical presentation.

Box 16. Points to Consider in Treating Diabetic Ketoacidosis

- A precipitating cause may be identified in 80% of patients.
- An ECG is indicated in all adult patients.
- Isotonic saline is initially preferred to rehydrate patients.
- Intravenous insulin is the preferred route of delivery.
- DKA patients are deplete in total-body potassium regardless of plasma potassium concentration.
- Bicarbonate should only be administered when specifically indicated.
- Preventing DKA is the long-term goal of good diabetes management.

Rehydration Process

Dehydration is present in almost all patients with DKA. There are many routes of water and/or electrolyte loss, including (1) polyuria, (2) hyperventilation, and (3) vomiting and diarrhea. The best index of the degree of dehydration is the magnitude of acute weight loss, which may be determined if the patient's baseline weight is known. Other clinical indices include orthostatic hypotension, dry mucous membranes, decreased tissue turgor, and thirst. A decrease in urine output is less reliable because of persistent osmotic diuresis with hyperglycemia. It is reasonable to assume an average weight loss of 5 to 10% of total body weight, or 3.5 to 7 liters of fluid in a 70-kilogram patient.

Adequate rehydration is extremely important in initial therapy because it helps restore and maintain the depleted vascular volume, and it enhances the kidney's ability to excrete glucose, thus lessening hyperglycemia.

Isotonic saline (0.9%) is usually the initial choice of rehydrating fluid. For patients who are hypertensive, hypernatremic, or at risk for congestive heart failure, a solution containing half (0.45%) isotonic saline may be preferable. In young children ($\leq$10 yr), calculate according to body surface area not weight (e.g., a 30-kg child has ~1 m^2 body surface area).

Box 17. Ketoacidosis Flow Sheet

Patient name ______________________ Patient wt (kg) ______________________

Admission date ______________________ Patient body surface area (m^2) ______________

	HOURS POSTADMISSION				
	0	**1**	**2**	**3**	**4**
THERAPY					
Fluid in (ml/h)	______	______	______	______	______
Fluid out (ml/h)	______	______	______	______	______
Insulin (U/h)	______	______	______	______	______
Potassium (meq/h)	______	______	______	______	______
Bicarbonate (meq/h)	______				
Phosphate (meq/h)	______	______	______	______	______
Glucose (g/h)	______	______	______	______	______
LABORATORY					
Glucose	______	______	______	______	______
pH	______		?		
Na^+	______		______	______	______
K^+	______		______	______	______
Cl^-	______	?	______	______	______
Bicarbonate	______	?	______	______	______
PO_4	______				______
Mg	______				______
Hct	______	?	?	?	?
Blood urea nitrogen	______				______
Creatinine	______				?
Calcium	______				
CLINICAL					
Mental status	______	______	______	______	______
Temperature	______	______	______	______	______
Pulse	______	______	______	______	______
Respiration	______	______	______	______	______
Blood pressure	______	______	______	______	______
ECG	______				
Weight (pre-DKA)	______				
Weight (postadmission)	______				

?, order if clinical situation warrants.
Other considerations are
type and cross match if necessary,
blood cultures if necessary,
aspirate stomach if comatose,
give oxygen if indicated, and
keep patient NPO.

Box 18. Fluid Replacement

HOUR 1

15 ml/kg isotonic NaCl (500 ml · m^{-2} · h^{-1}) (if elderly patient or one with heart disease, administer fluid cautiously, e.g., according to central venous pressure).

HOUR 2

Continue isotonic NaCl (15 ml/kg). However, if patient is hypernatremic, in congestive heart failure, or is a child, consider 0.5 isotonic sodium chloride.

HOUR 3

Reduce fluid rate to 7.5 ml · kg^{-1} · h^{-1}. Change fluid to 0.5 isotonic saline.

HOUR 4

Adjust fluid rate to meet clinical need. Consider rate of urine output in fluid replacement calculation.

When blood glucose approaches 300 mg/dl, change fluid to 5% dextrose in 0.5 isotonic saline. Continue intravenous fluids, *including insulin,* until acidosis is corrected and patient can ingest food without vomiting.

Then change to short-acting insulin subcutaneously every 4–6 h, giving first dose before discontinuing intravenous insulin.

Some specialists recommend intermediate-acting insulin so that a depot of insulin is available. Supplemental short-acting insulin is added as necessary, guided by blood glucose concentration.

Insulin Replacement

Because the cause of DKA in all patients includes absolute or relative insulin deficiency, *insulin must be provided.* Although rehydration by itself will reduce plasma nonesterified fatty acids and ketone bodies, insulin is required for suppression of ketoacid production and is thus necessary to correct acidosis. Insulin also inhibits glycogenolysis and gluconeogenesis, suppresses lipolysis, and facilitates sodium conservation by the kidney.

Only short-acting (regular) insulin should initially be used. Replacing insulin intravenously is the most direct route and is preferred if methods are available to regulate the infusion rate. Replacement via the intramuscular or subcutaneous routes has also been successful, so choice will depend on the clinical situation (Box 19). Intravenous therapy may be started with a bolus dose of insulin (0.15 U/kg) followed by insulin infusion at a rate of 0.1 U · kg^{-1} · h^{-1}.* This will bring about therapeutic insulin levels in almost all patients.

If no improvement in the acidosis as assessed by an increase in blood pH or bicarbonate or a decrease in the anion gap is apparent within 2 to 4 hours, the infusion rate should be doubled. If this fails to ameliorate acidosis, the clinician should consider events such as myocardial infarction or severe sepsis and should also consider obtaining consultation from a diabetologist.

The clinician should know that glucose is normalized more quickly than acidosis and that the insulin infusion should be continued until both are corrected. Therefore, when blood glucose approaches 300 mg/dl, the insulin infusion should be continued but at a reduced rate (about half) while 5% dextrose is added to the infusion so that blood glucose levels can be maintained at approximately 250 mg/dl for the first 12 to 24 hours.

Potassium Replacement

Patients with DKA are depleted in total-body potassium despite the fact that most have a normal or even elevated serum potassium level. The reasons for this are complex but include the catabolic state, potassium wasting in urine secondary to polyuria, inability of the kidney to rapidly conserve potassium and, often, the effects of vomiting and/or diarrhea.

Correct potassium replacement requires both caution and timely action. The following procedure is recommended. (1) Establish urine output to be certain the patient does not have renal failure. (2) Send blood samples to the laboratory to measure serum K^+. (3) Do an ECG to rapidly estimate if hypokalemia or hyperkalemia is present (high peaked T-waves in hyperkalemia;

*U · kg^{-1} · h^{-1} is often written U/(kg · h) or U/kg/h.

low T-waves with U-waves in hypokalemia). (4) Begin potassium replacement at the rate suggested in step 3. (5) When lab reports are available, alter rate if necessary (see Box 20 for suggested rates of replacement).

In most patients, once insulin infusion is begun, potassium replacement should be attended to promptly. Insulin tends to lower serum potassium by enhancing its movement back into cells. If potassium levels fall too low, hypokalemia-induced death from cardiac arrhythmia may result. Therefore, unless there is anuria, *the clinician should begin potassium replacement within 1 to 2 hours after starting insulin.* If there is anuria, estimation by ECG lead II is not appropriate; replacement must await a plasma potassium determination by the laboratory, and potassium should be infused with special caution.

Additional potassium may be needed if the patient is receiving sodium bicarbonate, because bicarbonate further enhances hypokalemia by promoting potassium movement back into cells.

Bicarbonate and Phosphate Replacement

Although it seems reasonable to administer sodium bicarbonate to the patient with DKA to correct the metabolic acidosis with alkali, it is not clear whether the potential benefits outweigh potential risks. The potential benefits of administering sodium bicarbonate include

- correcting extracellular acidosis,
- reducing excessive chloride administration,
- reducing respiratory rate and increasing comfort,
- reducing cardiac irritability, and
- increasing responsiveness of vascular system to pressor agents.

Potential harmful effects include

- *accelerated reduction in plasma potassium concentation,*
- sodium overload in elderly patients, and
- exacerbating intracellular acidosis.

For these reasons, routine bicarbonate administration is not recommended in most cases of DKA when pH is greater than or equal to 7.1. Some authorities still recommend administration of bicarbonate in patients with severe acidosis (i.e., pH <7.0), particularly when hypotension, shock, and arrhythmias are also present. Bicarbonate should only be given as an infusion of 1 to 2 meq/kg over 2 hours, and then the plasma bicarbonate level should be checked. The amount of bicarbonate administered should generally not exceed 3 meq/kg over 12 hours.

Patients presenting in DKA are usually phosphate depleted from a combination of decreased food intake, excessive catabolism, and increased urinary excretion. Furthermore, as with potassium, administering insulin enhances the movement of phosphate into cells, further reducing the plasma phosphate concentration.

There are pros and cons to administering phosphate, an ion important to many chemical reactions at the cellular

Box 19. Insulin Administration: Use Short-Acting (Regular) Insulin Only

Intravenous Route (preferred)

- Bolus dose 0.15 U/kg.
- Continuous infusion 0.1 U · kg^{-1} · h^{-1} (before connecting infusion tubing to patient, run 30 ml of insulin solution through tubing to saturate tubing adsorption sites).
- Changing insulin infusion rate
  - If no biochemical response is detected by 2–4 h, then double infusion rate (be sure to first check all infusion lines for patency).
  - If blood glucose declines below 300 mg/dl, then halve the infusion rate of insulin and add 5% dextrose (do not stop insulin infusion).
- Discontinuing infusion
  - Inject subcutaneous insulin.
  - One-half hour later, discontinue intravenous infusion.

Intramuscular or Subcutaneous Route (recommended only if no method is available to regulate intravenous insulin infusion rate)

- First hour of therapy, 0.5 U/kg.
- Each hour thereafter, 0.1 U/kg until blood glucose is reduced to 300 mg/dl.
- Every 2 h thereafter, inject 0.1 U/kg as necessary to maintain blood glucose concentration at 250 mg/dl. Some specialists recommend intermediate-acting insulin (outlined in Box 17).

Box 20. Potassium Replacement

- Initially, in patients with adequate urine output, ECG (lead II) may be used as a guide for plasma K^+ concentration.
- Replacement of K^+ is based on plasma K^+ concentration. If K^+ is
  - <3 meq/L, infuse 0.5 meq · kg^{-1} · h^{-1}
  - 3–4 meq/L, infuse 0.4 meq · kg^{-1} · h^{-1}
  - 4–5 meq/L, infuse 0.3 meq · kg^{-1} · h^{-1}
  - 5–6 meq/L, infuse 0.1–0.2 meq · kg^{-1} · h^{-1}
  - 6 meq/L, withhold until K^+ is <6.0 meq/L
- Add K^+ to replacement fluid therapy. If concentration of K^+ in infusate is 20–40 meq/L and infusion into peripheral vein causes irritation, infuse into central vein.
- Recheck plasma K^+ every 2 h if plasma concentration is <4 or >6 meq/L.
- Administer K^+ as K^+Cl^- or as potassium phosphate. However, do not exceed 90 meq/L potassium phosphate in 24 h because of danger of hypocalcemia.

level. One potential benefit is that hyperchloremia may be less likely to result when potassium is replaced as potassium phosphate instead of potassium chloride. However, administering too much phosphate can induce hypocalcemia. Therefore, calcium levels should be checked if phosphate is administered.

Although routine phosphate replacement has not been shown to be of benefit in treatment of diabetic ketoacidosis, conservative potassium phosphate administration, not to exceed 1.5 meq · kg^{-1} · 24 h^{-1}, is usually recommended for all patients. In this way, most of the potassium is administered as potassium chloride. More aggressive phosphate therapy should be considered in patients with an initial low phosphate concentration (≤2 meq/L) or rhabdomyolysis.

OTHER IMPORTANT CONSIDERATIONS

It is important to pursue other aspects of therapy while correcting the laboratory abnormalities. *First and foremost, the cause of DKA must be aggressively pursued* in both previously and newly diagnosed patients. Even if omission of an insulin injection by the patient is documented, the physician must be certain that there is no coexisting medical condition. In several reported series of patients admitted to the hospital with DKA, infection was the most common precipitating factor. Therefore, depending on clinical signs and symptoms, a chest X ray plus culture of the urine, throat, sputum, and blood may be warranted. Antibiotics should be considered in all cases of suspected infection. In adult patients an ECG is mandatory because myocardial infarction may precipitate DKA. As previously discussed, the clinician should also carefully investigate all possible causes of abdominal pain.

In addition to determination of the cause of DKA, *other supportive therapy must be considered.* Ensuring an airway and inserting a nasogastric tube to drain gastric contents in comatose patients are strongly recommended to prevent aspiration pneumonia. Low-dose subcutaneous heparin (5000 U every 12 h) is often recommended to prevent hypercoagulability, especially in elderly patients. However, data proving its efficacy are lacking.

Be alert to complications of treatment. Potential complications directly attributable to the treatment of DKA must be anticipated.

- Generally, glucose will be normalized more quickly than acidosis. Premature discontinuation of insulin may result in persistence and worsening of ketoacidosis.
- Too aggressive fluid replacement (particularly with isotonic saline) may induce congestive heart failure. Therefore, frequent auscultation of the lungs is mandatory.
- Nausea and vomiting from feeding the patient before gastric peristalsis has returned can result in aspiration pneumonia. Therefore, solid foods should be introduced cautiously.
- Hypoglycemia can occur if the insulin infusion is not supplemented with glucose when the blood glucose concentration is less than 300 mg/dl. If acidosis is still present, the insulin infusion must be continued at 0.05 to

$0.1\ U \cdot kg^{-1} \cdot h^{-1}$, and glucose must be infused to maintain the blood glucose concentration above 200 mg/dl.

- Finally, cerebral edema and death may occur, particularly in children. Although the etiology of this complication has not been determined, some authorities believe that it is caused by correcting hyperglycemia too rapidly.

Therefore, the blood glucose concentration should be maintained at approximately 250 mg/dl during the first 12 to 24 hours of therapy.

Intermediate Patient Care

As the patient improves, the question of when to discontinue intravenous insulin and fluids and begin subcutaneous insulin will arise. To answer this question, several clinical parameters must be considered. First, is the patient clinically stable with normal vital signs? Second, has the patient's blood pH, plasma bicarbonate level, or anion gap returned toward normal levels (i.e., has the acidosis been corrected)? Third, can the patient drink fluids without experiencing nausea and vomiting? Fourth, has the precipitating stress (e.g., infection) been controlled? If the answer to any of the above questions is no, then the physician should probably continue intravenous insulin and fluid.

When subcutaneous insulin is begun, several points should be kept in mind. First, because subcutaneous insulin takes effect more slowly than intravenous insulin loses its effectiveness, the first subcutaneous insulin injection should be given 15 to 30 minutes before termination of the intravenous insulin infusion. This initial dose should be approximately 0.2 U/kg, and blood glucose should be checked every 4 to 6 hours to determine whether an increase or a decrease in insulin is needed. Second, some clinicians prefer to use short-acting insulin only, in divided doses (0.1–0.25 U/kg) every 4 to 6 hours for the first 24 hours, before beginning a regimen with a longer-acting insulin such as NPH or lente. Short-acting insulin permits rapid adjustment of the insulin dose to control blood glucose during this transition phase. Other authorities recommend the use of intermediate-acting insulin (0.2 U/kg) from the outset to prevent recurrence of acidosis in the transition phase. Third, the patient may remain mildly insulin resistant for several weeks, so the dose of subcutaneous insulin may exceed the patient's usual requirements.

PREVENTIVE CARE

Most often, DKA can be prevented, given appropriate patient education and prompt physician attention. Patients must learn to contact their physicians as soon as they become ill, have nausea and vomiting, fever, or persistent hyperglycemia or hyperketonuria. When contacted early, the physician is often able to treat DKA successfully by prescribing frequent injections of short-acting insulin and by oral administration of fluids. It may also be possible to rehydrate and reinsulinize the patient in the doctor's office or emergency room, thereby preventing progression to DKA and expensive hospitalization.

However, when there is any doubt that the patient can be successfully treated in the emergency room, hospitalization is indicated. *For patients who have repeated episodes of DKA,* psychological consultation should be considered. Many of these patients, especially adolescents, may use the hospital as a haven from social and psychological pressures.

CONCLUSION

The pathophysiology of DKA can now be understood in the context of insulin deficiency and excessive counterregulatory hormones combining their effects to produce a severe state of life-threatening metabolic decompensation. Insulin, fluids, and electrolytes, given judiciously under appropriate guidelines in a hospital setting, form the cornerstone of treatment. A precipitating event such as infection, infarction, or deliberate omission of insulin must be identified and treated.

BIBLIOGRAPHY

Foster DW, McGarry JD: The metabolic derangements and treatment of diabetic ketoacidosis. *N Engl J Med* 309:159–69, 1983

Keller U: Diabetic ketoacidosis: current views of pathogenesis and treatment. *Diabetologia* 29:71–77, 1986

Kreisberg RA: Diabetic ketoacidosis: new concepts and trends in pathogenesis and treatment. *Ann Intern Med* 88:681–95, 1978

Schade DS, Eaton RP, Alberti KGMM, Johnston DG: *Diabetic Coma.* Albuquerque, Univ. of New Mexico Press, 1981

Sperling MA: Diabetic ketoacidosis. *Pediatr Clin N Am* 31:591–610, 1984

Hypoglycemia

INTRODUCTION

The precise blood glucose level at which patients develop symptoms of hypoglycemia is difficult to define but, generally, symptoms do not occur until blood glucose is less than 50 to 60 mg/dl. Clinical hypoglycemia is the occurrence of typical adrenergic and/or neuroglycopenic symptoms with low blood glucose levels. Because of its sporadic and somewhat unpredictable nature and because of the need for rapid treatment, hypoglycemia is often self-diagnosed on the basis of predominantly adrenergic symptoms and may be treated without documentation of the blood glucose level.

HYPOGLYCEMIA: MILD, MODERATE, AND SEVERE

Insulin reactions, or hypoglycemia, can be conveniently classified into three categories: mild, moderate, and severe.

Symptoms of Mild Reactions

Mild reactions usually consist of tremors, palpitations, sweating, and excessive hunger. These symptoms are mostly mediated through the autonomic (adrenergic) nervous system. Cognitive deficits usually do not accompany mild reactions, and patients are capable of self-treatment. These mild symptoms respond within 10 to 15 minutes to oral ingestion of 10 to 15 grams of simple carbohydrate.

Symptoms of Moderate Reactions

Moderate reactions include neuroglycopenic as well as adrenergic symptoms, e.g., headache, mood changes, irritability, decreased attentiveness, and drowsiness. Because of confusion, impaired judgment, and/or weakness, patients may require assistance in treating themselves. Moderate reactions produce longer-lasting and somewhat more severe symptoms and often require a second dose of simple carbohydrate.

Symptoms of Severe Reactions

Severe reactions are characterized by unresponsiveness, unconsciousness, or convulsions. Approximately 10% of insulin-dependent (type I) patients suffer one severe reaction each year, which will require emergency measures such as parenteral glucagon or intravenous glucose.

Potential Effects of Hypoglycemia

Mild hypoglycemia is usually only a nuisance. It can cause hunger with consequent overeating, thus contributing to obesity or hyperglycemia.

In contrast, moderate and severe reactions may be seriously disabling in many ways, and blood glucose should be kept high enough to avoid them. Hypoglycemia that interferes with normal thinking makes taking a school examination an impossible task; riding a bicycle, driving a car, or operating dangerous machinery becomes potentially disastrous. Repeated or prolonged episodes may cause irreparable damage to the central nervous system, especially in very young children. Finally, such reactions should be avoided because of their deleterious effects on the morale of the patient and family members.

Some patients develop either a phobic fear of hypoglycemia or an inappropriate lack of concern. Fear of hypoglycemia can lead to chronic overeating or undertreatment with insulin, or both. Maintaining blood glucose levels of 240 to 400 mg/dl to avoid hypoglycemia increases the risk of metabolic complications, including diabetic ketoacidosis. In contrast, patients with a nonchalant attitude toward hypoglycemic reactions may maintain levels of blood glucose that are too low and will consequently be at greater risk for recurrent severe hypoglycemia. These patients can sometimes be identified by their near-normal glycohemoglobin levels.

Antecedents of Severe Hypoglycemia

Certain circumstances favor development of prolonged, incapacitating, and occasionally life-threatening hypoglycemia. Patients with "hypoglycemic unawareness" are always at increased risk for severe reactions. The counterregulatory hormone response to hypoglycemia and the adrenergic symptoms tend to decrease after several years of diabetes so that neuroglycopenic symptoms become the first manifestation for many patients. Beta blockers and intensive insulin therapy may also diminish early warning signs.

Delaying treatment is another common reason that mild hypoglycemia becomes more severe. Because early adrenergic warning signs like headache, hunger, mood or behavior changes, or weakness are not specific to hypoglycemia, they are frequently misinterpreted or overlooked. This is especially likely if the patient's attention is directed elsewhere, which may occur during strenuous activity. Hypoglycemia during sleep is particularly difficult to detect; family members should be alert to unusual sounds or activity during the patient's sleep.

Box 21. Common Causes of Hypoglycemia

Insulin errors (inadvertent or deliberate)
- reversal of morning and evening dosage
- reversal of short- and intermediate-acting insulin
- improper timing of insulin in relation to food
- excessive insulin dosage

Erratic or altered absorption of insulin
- more rapid absorption from exercising limbs
- unpredictable absorption from hypertrophied injection sites

Use of more purified insulin preparations or change from mixed species to single species or human insulin

Diet
- omitted or inadequate amounts of food
- timing errors: late snacks or meals

Exercise
- unplanned activity
- prolonged duration or increased intensity of activity

Alcohol and drugs
- impaired hepatic gluconeogenesis associated with alcohol intake
- impaired mentation associated with alcohol, marijuana, and cocaine

COMMON CAUSES OF HYPOGLYCEMIA

The factors precipitating an episode of hypoglycemia can often be identified by looking back over the events of several hours preceding the reaction (see Box 21 for the most common causes).

Inadvertent or deliberate *errors in insulin dose* are a frequent cause of hypoglycemia; other causes are *changes in timing or schedule* of insulin administration or meals. For example, sleeping later than usual is potentially dangerous for patients taking insulin because it disrupts the balance and timing between insulin and food. *Changing insulin type* to a more highly purified (and possibly more potent) preparation or from a mixed-species insulin to a purified pork or human insulin can cause hypoglycemia because of more rapid absorption or other factors.

Vigorous unexpected *exercise* or activity ("burst" activity) is commonly associated with hypoglycemia. Aerobic exercise of prolonged duration or increased intensity can cause a reaction that occurs several hours after the activity period ends or even the next day.

Alcohol, marijuana, or other drugs often mask a patient's awareness of hypoglycemia in its earliest stages. By inhibiting the liver's gluconeogenic capacity, alcohol also prevents the body's normal ability to provide glucose and restore low glucose levels toward normal. Some of the most severe hypoglycemic reactions occur during or after parties because the combination of physical activity and the use of alcohol or drugs can mask recognition of the problem and prevent the usual self-correction of hypoglycemia.

Anticipating and Preventing Hypoglycemia

Once a situation that leads to hypoglycemia is identified, adjustments can often be made to prevent future episodes.

Sleeping Late

Although most patients can safely sleep an extra 30 to 45 minutes without particular adjustments, patients who oversleep more than 45 minutes need to plan in advance to alter insulin or food intake. For example, if sleeping late is anticipated, a 10 to 15% reduction of intermediate- or long-acting insulin on the previous evening is an effective means of preventing hypoglycemia. When the patient awakens, the entire day's schedule of insulin and meals is advanced in time. Even the next day's schedule may be affected. *All patients should be cautioned against awakening and taking insulin without eating and then resuming sleep.* However, awakening early, performing a blood glucose test, administering insulin, eating breakfast, and then going back to sleep is generally safe. Patients treated with intensive therapy to achieve near-normal blood glucose levels may not have as much flexibility as conventionally treated patients.

Exercise

To compensate for increased caloric needs of exercise, increased absorption of insulin from exercising muscles, and increased insulin sensitivity induced by extra activity, several strategies to prevent hypoglycemia can be employed. Most important, the exercising patient should always have a source of short-acting carbohydrate immediately available.

If early signs of hypoglycemia develop during exercise, the exercise should be halted and an appropriate amount of carbohydrate eaten (see p. 58). On the other hand, if similar exercise has previously resulted in hypoglycemia, patients can anticipate and prevent it by snacking before, during, or after exercise, depending on when the episode occurred. Decisions regarding the type and time of extra food can be made based on self-monitoring of blood glucose (SMBG).

Alternatively, hypoglycemia can be prevented by anticipatory adjustments of insulin. For example, if a patient usually takes short-acting (regular) insulin before breakfast but is planning to exercise after breakfast, the insulin dose can be reduced by 10 to 20%. This strategy may be preferable for patients who do not want to increase the size of a meal before exercise or who are overweight.

Role of SMBG

The availability of SMBG has made the detection and treatment of hypoglycemia practical, even in the subclinical range. Therefore, SMBG should be taught to patients with frequent hypoglycemia who do not already use it, and its frequency should be increased in patients who do. Changes in insulin injection, eating or exercise schedules, travel, and other activities recognized as contributors to hypoglycemia call for increased frequency of monitoring. Patients should be instructed to treat asymptomatic hypoglycemia detected by SMBG.

TREATMENT

Mild Hypoglycemic Reactions

For mild reactions, 10 to 15 grams of simple oral carbohydrate work quickly to raise the blood glucose and stop classic symptoms. Four to 6 ounces of carbohydrate-containing liquids (e.g., unsweetened fruit juices, carbonated drinks), five to six Lifesavers, one tablespoon of honey or Karo syrup, four teaspoons or packets of granulated sugar, or six ½-inch sugar cubes all provide sufficient short-acting carbohydrate to terminate mild reactions. Hypoglycemic reactions that occur during the night should be treated initially with 10 to 15 grams of carbohydrate followed by a longer-acting mixture of carbohydrate and protein, e.g., 8 ounces of milk or 4 ounces of milk and a few crackers. This is intended to prevent further hypoglycemia during the night.

Commercially available glucose tablets have the added benefit of being premeasured to help prevent overtreatment. Glucose gel products or small tubes of cake frosting are convenient for children or patients who are uncooperative when hypoglycemic. Chocolate and ice cream should be avoided for treating acute hypoglycemia because the fat content could retard absorption of available sugar and could contribute to obesity from ingestion of unnecessary calories.

Because there is always a risk that mild hypoglycemia will progress to a more severe reaction, all episodes must be treated promptly. Patients should be instructed never to continue driving when they begin to experience hypoglycemia. They should stop, treat the hypoglycemia, and wait 10 to 15 minutes for full recovery before they resume driving.

Moderate Hypoglycemia

Individuals with moderate reactions will often respond to the oral carbohydrates listed previously but may require more than one treatment and take longer to fully recover. These patients may be alert but will frequently be uncooperative or belligerent. Under such circumstances, if it becomes difficult to cajole the patient to take an oral carbohydrate, administration of glucagon may be more appropriate.

Severe Hypoglycemia

Patients with impaired consciousness or an inability to swallow may aspirate and should rarely be treated with oral carbohydrate. *These patients require either glucagon or intravenous glucose.* If these are not available, glucose gel products, applied between the patient's cheek and gum, may be of some help.

Generally, clinical improvement should occur within 10 to 15 minutes after glucagon injection and within 1 to 5 minutes of intravenous glucose administration. However, if hypoglycemia was prolonged or extremely severe, complete recovery of normal mental function may not return for hours. Repeated boluses of intravenous glucose do not hasten recovery unless blood glucose measurements show persistent hypoglycemia. If the hypoglycemic event was associated with convulsions, the postictal period may be associated with severe headache, lethargy, amnesia, or vomiting. Decreased muscle control may also be seen and requires medical evaluation if it persists. Recurrent episodes of severe hypoglycemia can lead to permanent cognitive deficits. To prevent recurrence, patients should eat their planned meals or snacks (~10% of daily calories) after initial treatment of moderate or severe reactions or when treating any nocturnal reaction.

Glucagon

The dose of glucagon needed to treat moderate or severe hypoglycemia for a child under the age of 5 years is 0.25 to 0.50 milligram; for an older child (5–10 yr), 0.50 to 1 milligram; and for those over 10 years of age, 1 milligram. Glucagon should be given intramuscularly or subcutaneously in the deltoid or anterior thigh region. Parents, roommates, and spouses should be taught how to mix, draw up, and administer glucagon so that they are properly prepared for emergency situations. Kits that include a syringe prefilled with diluting fluid are available.

Intravenous Glucose

If medical staff and equipment are available, intravenous glucose should be given as a primary treatment in preference to glucagon. The usual dose is 10 to 25 grams administered as 50% dextrose over 1 to 3 minutes. The dose can be titrated according to the patient's response. After the bolus injection, intravenous glucose (5–10 g/h) should be continued until the patient has fully recovered and is able to eat.

HYPOGLYCEMIA WITH REBOUND HYPERGLYCEMIA

Hypoglycemia followed by "rebound" hyperglycemia, also called the Somogyi phenomenon, may complicate diabetes management in several ways (Box 22). The phenomenon originates during hypoglycemia, with the secretion of counterregulatory hormones (glucagon,

Box 22. When to Suspect Rebound Hyperglycemia

- Unstable glucose results characterized by daily fluctuations between hypoglycemia and severe hyperglycemia
- Increasing glucose levels despite increasing insulin doses
- Awakening with ketonuria in the absence of glycosuria
- Awakening with headaches, restless sleep, nightmares, or enuresis (all suggestive of nocturnal hypoglycemia); nausea or vomiting without explanation
- High insulin doses
  - children: $>1.0\ U \cdot kg^{-1} \cdot day^{-1}$*
  - adolescents: $>1.5\ U \cdot kg^{-1} \cdot day^{-1}$
  - adults: $>1.5\ U \cdot kg^{-1} \cdot day^{-1}$

*Alternate notation: U/(kg · day) or U/kg/day.

epinephrine, growth hormone, and cortisol). This hormonal surge, together with falling insulin levels, leaves counterregulatory hormones relatively unopposed. Hepatic glucose production is stimulated, thereby raising blood glucose levels excessively. These hormones may cause insulin resistance for a 12- to 48-hour period.

The frequency of this phenomenon is debated. It usually follows nocturnal hypoglycemia, but it may occur after hypoglycemia that occurs at any time. The hypoglycemic event that precedes the rebound may or may not produce sufficient symptoms to make it recognizable.

If rebound hyperglycemia goes unrecognized and insulin dosage is increased, a cycle of overinsulinization may result, i.e., more hypoglycemia, more rebound hyperglycemia, more insulin, more hypoglycemia. As a general rule, when hyperglycemia does not respond as expected to treatment adjustments, undetected hypoglycemia and rebound hyperglycemia should be considered as a possible explanation. Instead of increasing insulin dosage day after day, the clinician who suspects rebound hyperglycemia should endeavor to detect (via SMBG) and avoid the initiating hypoglycemic event.

Nocturnal rebound hyperglycemia should be investigated by measuring blood glucose levels between 0200 and 0400 h and again at 0700 h. If blood glucose levels between 0200 and 0400 h are less than 50 to 60 mg/dl and those at 0700 h are more than 180 to 200 mg/dl, rebound hyperglycemia may have occurred. A decrease in presupper intermediate-acting insulin or its deferral to approximately 2100 h or an appropriate change in bedtime snack should prevent nocturnal hypoglycemia.

CONCLUSION

Severe hypoglycemia can be life threatening if not treated promptly. Even mild and moderate hypoglycemia can cause both short- and long-term problems. All patients should be taught to be aware of the signs of hypoglycemia and should be encouraged to use SMBG more frequently to prevent and monitor episodes. All families should be taught how to use glucagon and when to call for medical assistance.

BIBLIOGRAPHY

Cryer PE, Gerich JE: Glucose counterregulation, hypoglycemia and intensive insulin therapy in diabetes mellitus. *N Engl J Med* 313:232–41, 1985

Gale EAM, Tattersall RB: Unrecognized nocturnal hypoglycaemia in insulin-treated diabetics. *Lancet* 9:1049–52, 1979

Havlin CE, Cryer PE: Nocturnal hypoglycemia does not commonly result in major morning hyperglycemia in patients with diabetes mellitus. *Diabetes Care* 2:141–47, 1987

Simonson DC, Tamborlane WV, DeFronzo RA, Sherwin RS: Intensive insulin therapy reduces counterregulatory hormone response to hypoglycemia in patients with type I diabetes. *Ann Intern Med* 103:184–90, 1985

Pregnancy

INTRODUCTION

Insulin-dependent (type I) diabetes mellitus complicates approximately 0.1 to 0.5% of all pregnancies. During the past decade and a half, perinatal outcome has improved remarkably in this high-risk group. Except for deaths due to major fetal malformations, the perinatal mortality rate for women with diabetes who receive optimal care now approaches that of the general obstetric population.

Management of the patient with type I diabetes during pregnancy ideally involves an experienced health-care team, including the internist or diabetologist, obstetrician or maternal-fetal specialist, pediatrician or neonatologist, teaching nurse, dietitian, the patient herself, and her partner. Experience indicates that the outcome for both mother and baby is generally more favorable when an experienced team is responsible for management during pregnancy, delivery, and the perinatal period. When a team is not conveniently available, phone consultation with individual specialists is helpful.

Pregnant women are usually highly motivated; therefore, this time is ideal for teaching self-care skills they can use for the rest of their lives.

RISK FACTORS

What factors help quantify maternal and fetal risk in the diabetic pregnancy? Generally, risk factors fall into two categories: those relating to diabetes and its control and those relating to vascular complications. Thus, pregnancies complicated by type I diabetes can be divided into two groups: women with diabetes, and women with diabetes *and* vascular complications.

Diabetes and Its Control

The earlier the onset of diabetes and the longer its duration, the worse the prognosis for good perinatal outcome. The quality of maternal glucose control throughout pregnancy is also an important consideration. Ketoacidosis and associated intrauterine deaths are most common in patients with poor blood glucose control.

Vasculopathy

The greater the degree of vasculopathy, the greater the likelihood of a poor outcome for mother and child. *Nephropathy,* particularly if associated with hypertension, appears to bring the greatest hazards, increasing the risk of preeclampsia, fetal growth retardation, and preterm delivery. Pregnancy can contribute to a worsening of *retinal disease* in women with background or proliferative retinopathy, especially in the presence of hypertension; women with active proliferative retinopathy are at greatest risk for loss of visual acuity. Maternal deaths have been reported in patients with *coronary artery disease.*

Other prognostically bad signs during pregnancy include ketoacidosis, pyelonephritis, preeclampsia, and poor clinic attendance or neglect.

MATERNAL METABOLISM DURING PREGNANCY

During gestation, maternal metabolism adapts to provide the fetus with an uninterrupted supply of fuel. Normal pregnancy is characterized by maternal hyperinsulinemia and insulin resistance, changes induced by hormones of pregnancy that are most marked late in gestation.

In nondiabetic women, estrogen and progesterone directly alter maternal islet cell function, producing beta-cell hyperplasia and contributing to maternal hyperinsulinemia. In addition, maternal cortisol is elevated during pregnancy, which potentiates glucose intolerance. Human placental lactogen (hPL), a growth hormone–like protein synthesized by the placental syncytiotrophoblast, produces insulin resistance and augments maternal lipolysis. As placental mass enlarges during pregnancy, hPL levels rise, allowing increased maternal utilization of fats for energy and sparing of glucose for fetal consumption. In late pregnancy, the progression of overnight maternal fasting ketosis is so accelerated that delaying breakfast may result in significant ketonuria.

In the pregnancy complicated by diabetes, periods of maternal hyperglycemia produce fetal hyperglycemia. Larger amounts of maternal amino acids and other fuels also cross to the fetus. Elevated levels of maternal glucose and other nutrients stimulate the fetal pancreas, resulting in beta-cell hyperplasia and hyperinsulinemia. This combination of fetal overnutrition and fetal hyperinsulinemia contributes to the morbidity and mortality observed in the infant of the diabetic mother.

CARE BEFORE CONCEPTION

Treatment of the patient with type I diabetes must begin *before* gestation (Box 23). For this reason, any regular visit to the physician by a reproductive-age woman, *from teenage* to middle age, should be considered a preconception visit. These contacts provide an important opportunity to discuss the patient's contraceptive needs and her thoughts and concerns about a future pregnancy and to establish a data base that can be used in assessing perinatal risk (Box 24). Adolescents in particular should be encouraged to discuss these issues routinely with members of the health-care team.

Important periodic assessments include measurement of blood pressure, an ophthalmologic examination, an electrocardiogram, and a 24-hour urine collection for creatinine clearance and protein excretion. Glycosylated hemoglobin should be performed routinely, and self-monitoring of blood glucose (SMBG) taught, if needed.

Immune status against rubella should also be checked before conception. Consultation with a nutritionist and a review of the patient's exercise program are important. The patient must understand that smoking and alcohol are strictly prohibited during pregnancy.

Because the pregnancy complicated by type I diabetes may cause emotional and financial stress, it is essential to evaluate the psychosocial interactions of the patient and her partner, their support network, and their financial resources.

CONGENITAL MALFORMATIONS: RISK AND DETECTION

The incidence of major congenital malformations is increased three- to fourfold in the offspring of patients with type I diabetes over the 2 to 3% in the general population. Incidence increases to 20 to 25% among women with markedly elevated glycosylated hemoglobin in the first trimester.

Steadily accumulating evidence links such malformations with inadequate diabetes control during embryogenesis (gestational weeks 3–7). For this reason, patients should be as near normoglycemic as possible at the time of conception and throughout the first trimester. All women of childbearing age should be made aware of these risks, and if pregnancy is considered, they should be encouraged to use contraception until excellent glycemic control is achieved (see **Philosophy and Goals**). The risk of fetal anomalies should be reviewed at the first prenatal visit.

Many fetal anomalies, particularly in the central nervous system, heart, skeleton, and urinary tract, may be detected before birth. The evaluation for a potential fetal malformation should include a maternal serum alpha-fetoprotein level at 16 weeks, a detailed

Box 23. Care Before Conception

- Discuss contraceptive program
- Establish data base for perinatal risk
  - Assess vascular status:
    - ophthalmologic examination
    - ECG
    - 24-h urine for protein
    - creatinine clearance
    - check all peripheral pulses
  - Assess glycemic control via glycohemoglobin
- Optimize glycemic control; teach SMBG if needed
- Refer for assessment of nutritional adequacy; adjust if needed
- Determine immune status against rubella
- Evaluate psychosocial setting
- Other
  - Caution patient against smoking or excessive alcohol
  - Assess exercise program

Box 24. Preconception Counseling: Common Questions and Answers

- Q. How will pregnancy affect my life expectancy?

  A. Pregnancy is not generally life threatening, but serious complications can occur. There is no evidence that pregnancy shortens the lives of women with type I diabetes, except for those with established coronary artery disease. However, diabetic women do face a higher risk for certain complications. If ketoacidosis occurs, it is likely to be more dangerous during pregnancy; and both preeclampsia and delivery by cesarean section are more common in diabetic women.

- Q. What effect will pregnancy have on diabetic nephropathy?

  A. There is no evidence that pregnancy will permanently worsen diabetic nephropathy, although a temporary increase in proteinuria and decrease in creatinine clearance may occur. On the other hand, advanced nephropathy may jeopardize both mother and infant. Severe diabetic nephropathy may increase the likelihood of early delivery and/or a smaller-than-normal infant. Factors that point in this direction include
  - proteinuria >3 g/24 h in the 1st trimester or >10 g/24 h in the 3rd trimester,
  - serum creatinine >1.5 mg/dl at the start of pregnancy,
  - hematocrit <25% in the 3rd trimester, and
  - hypertension.

- Q. What effect will pregnancy have on diabetic retinopathy?

  A. Except for women with active proliferative retinopathy, pregnancy is usually an ophthalmologically stable period. Women without diabetic retinopathy will not usually develop it during pregnancy. Very few women with background retinopathy present at the start of pregnancy may experience some worsening of this condition but very rarely to a proliferative stage. Proliferative retinopathy treated by laser photocoagulation and stable before pregnancy will generally remain so. In contrast, many women with active proliferative retinopathy that has not been treated with photocoagulation experience a serious worsening of this complication during pregnancy.

- Q. Will the baby develop diabetes mellitus?

  A. Although the infant is slightly more likely to develop type I diabetes, the risk is not very high—approximately 2% during the first 20 years of life.

- Q. Can I use birth control pills?

  A. Young women without vascular complications may use a low-dose estrogen/progestin oral contraceptive. Those with hypertension or vasculopathy should use a progestin-only pill (or some other means of birth control).

- Q. What effect will diabetes have on the baby?

  A. The answer to this question appears to hinge largely on the mother's blood glucose control; generally, the better the diabetes control, the fewer the complications. In the first weeks of pregnancy, poor diabetes control seems to increase the occurrence of fetal malformations. Later, high blood glucose levels may bring about other serious consequences. Because glucose crosses from the mother to the fetus but insulin does not, high maternal glucose stimulates the *fetus* to overproduce insulin, which may
  - cause excessive fetal growth,
  - prevent the baby's lungs (and other organs) from maturing at a normal pace, or
  - give the baby serious hypoglycemia after birth, when it no longer receives glucose from the mother.

  In addition, high glucose levels are associated with sudden unexplained fetal death late in pregnancy.

ultrasound examination of fetal anatomy at 16 to 18 weeks, and an assessment of fetal cardiac structure by echocardiography at 20 weeks (Box 25). All of these studies require interpretation by individuals experienced in prenatal diagnosis.

MATERNAL GLUCOSE CONTROL DURING PREGNANCY

It is generally accepted that excellent control of maternal diabetes will reduce the risks of fetal demise, excessive fetal growth, and delayed pulmonary maturation. During a nondiabetic pregnancy, maternal plasma glucose rarely exceeds 100 mg/dl, ranging from fasting levels of 60 mg/dl to postprandial levels of 120 mg/dl. These values should be the therapeutic objectives for pregnancies complicated by type I diabetes (Table 14).

Maintaining maternal glucose levels in this range throughout gestation is difficult. During the first trimester, when morning sickness may be troublesome, the risk of hypoglycemia is increased; hypoglycemia is most likely during the night, when the mother is fasting but the fetus and placenta continue to consume glucose. In contrast, during the early third trimester, when the diabetogenic stress of pregnancy is greatest, insulin needs may rise 50% over 4 to 6 weeks, heightening the risk for ketoacidosis.

Monitoring Control

SMBG

During pregnancy, women with type I diabetes must use SMBG to assess control. SMBG has been shown to decrease the need for hospitalization and reduce the cost of care. Patients should monitor in the fasting state, before each meal, and possibly 1 to 2 hours after meals. Testing at 0200 to 0300 h is necessary for patients who are likely to experience nocturnal hypoglycemia, those who have persistent fasting hyperglycemia, or those who are using continuous subcutaneous insulin-infusion (CSII) pump treatment. The patient should be instructed to maintain a careful record of her daily glucose values with comments about calorie intake and exercise.

Available data are too limited to permit specific recommendations regarding exercise programs in pregnant women with diabetes.

Box 25. Fetal Evaluation

MIDPREGNANCY (16–20 wk): to detect fetal anomalies

- Maternal serum alpha-fetoprotein
- Ultrasonography
- Fetal echocardiography

LATE PREGNANCY (28 wk to delivery): to assess fetal well-being

- Maternal assessment of fetal activity
- Nonstress test
- Contraction stress test
- Fetal biophysical profile
- Ultrasonography
- Lecithin-to-sphingomyelin (L/S) ratio, lung profile

Glycoslated Hemoglobin

A glycosylated hemoglobin determination should be obtained at the patient's first prenatal visit to assess previous glycemic control. This test should be repeated at least once every 3 months (see **Philosophy and Goals**).

Urine Testing

Although the increased glomerular filtration rate of pregnancy limits the value of urinary glucose testing, patients should be instructed to test urine for ketones before breakfast every day and if capillary glucose levels exceed 200 mg/dl.

Insulin Regimen During Pregnancy

An insulin regimen tailored to the patient's needs can be developed based on SMBG data, the meal plan, and the exercise regimen. Most women will require *at least* two daily injections of a mixture of intermediate-acting (NPH, lente) and short-acting (regular) insulins. Patients usually receive two-thirds of the total insulin dose at breakfast and the remaining third at supper. The morning combination ordinarily contains twice as much intermediate-acting as short-acting insulin, and the evening dose is divided equally between the two.

Table 14. Target Blood Glucose Levels in Pregnancy

TIME OF MEASUREMENT	BLOOD GLUCOSE (mg/dl)
Before breakfast	60–90
Before lunch, supper, and bedtime snack	60–105
2 h after meals	≤120
0200–0600 h	>60

Glycosylated hemoglobin levels should be within the normal range for the individual laboratory.

Delaying the evening intermediate-acting component until near bedtime may help to avoid glycemic irregularities overnight. In this case, the morning injection remains the same, but short-acting insulin alone is given at supper and intermediate-acting insulin alone at bedtime. Postponing the intermediate-acting component decreases the likelihood of the Somogyi phenomenon (hypoglycemia followed by rebound hyperglycemia) as well as the dawn phenomenon (waning of the insulin effect in the early-morning hours leading to prebreakfast hyperglycemia). (See **Hypoglycemia,** p. 74, for more on rebound hyperglycemia.)

Some patients prefer the flexibility of a four-injection regimen: short-acting insulin at breakfast, lunch, and supper, with an injection of intermediate- or long-acting (ultralente) insulin at bedtime.

In general, if glucose levels remain elevated, the corresponding insulin dose is increased by 20%.

CSII Therapy

Selected patients who have used CSII pump therapy before gestation may be continued on this program. However, CSII treatment appears to offer no significant advantage over multiple insulin injections and may actually increase risk. The nocturnal basal infusion dose must often be decreased to reduce the risk of hypoglycemia, and ketoacidosis and intrauterine fetal death can occur in association with pump failure or maternal infection.

NUTRITION NEEDS

The daily nutrition needs of pregnant women with type I diabetes include approximately 30 to 35 kcal/kg of desired pregnant body weight. Approximately 20% of the calories should be derived from protein, 30% from fats, and 50% from carbohydrates.

For most patients, 10% of the calories should be consumed at breakfast, 30% at lunch, and 30% at supper. The remaining 30% of calories should be distributed among several snacks, particularly a bedtime snack to decrease the risk of nocturnal hypoglycemia. Additional snacks may be added if the patient anticipates an increase in exercise. Patients with persistently elevated mid-morning glucose levels should reduce the calorie content of breakfast and redistribute the calories to lunch and supper. The presence of morning ketonuria with normal glucose levels indicates the need to increase the calorie content of the bedtime snack or to consider adding an 0300 h snack. The calorie content of the meal plan may be reduced in women who are obese, who demonstrate early excessive weight gain, or who have a sedentary life-style. In such patients, weight maintenance, rather than actual weight loss, should be the aim. A daily meal plan of 25 kcal/kg ideal prepregnancy body weight should achieve this goal. Patterns of weight gain and recommended calorie needs for women who begin pregnancy at below, average, or above ideal weight can be obtained from appropriate references (also see **Nutrition,** Table 9).

OUTPATIENT CARE

Most women with type I diabetes may be managed as outpatients throughout gestation. Some may benefit from early hospitalization to evaluate cardiovascular and renal status and glucose control. In addition, failure to maintain acceptable glucose levels, worsening hypertension, or infectious complications such as a viral illness or pyelonephritis may necessitate hospitalization. A urine culture should be ordered in the first trimester.

Clinic visits can be scheduled at 1- to 2-week intervals for most women. At each visit, the patient's SMBG log should be reviewed, problems with hyperglycemia and/or hypoglycemia discussed, and the patient's weight gain and blood pressure checked. The patient should also be instructed to telephone the physician promptly if there are any episodes of hypoglycemia (<50 mg/dl) or hyperglycemia (>200 mg/dl) so that appropriate remedial action may be taken.

Throughout gestation, the physician directing the patient's management must communicate regularly with other members of the health-care team. If background retinopathy has been detected, repeat ophthalmologic examinations should be obtained in the second or third trimester; proliferative retinopathy requires more intensive follow-up. In patients with nephropathy, renal function studies including creatinine clearance and protein excretion should be repeated in each trimester.

Assessment of Fetal Condition

Significant advances have been made in the ability to assess fetal growth and well-being. The detection of fetal malformations between 16 and 20 weeks is discussed on p. 77. In the third trimester, attention should be directed toward the assessment of fetal well-being, growth, and pulmonary maturation (Box 25). Several approaches should be used to assess fetal condition to prevent sudden intrauterine death, a catastrophe most likely to occur during the final 4 to 6 weeks of gestation.

Patient Self-Assessment

Maternal monitoring of fetal activity has proved to be a simple yet valuable screening approach in high-risk pregnancies. Daily assessment of fetal movement may be started at 28 weeks gestation. The patient counts fetal activity for several 30- to 60-minute periods throughout the day or records the time of day at which she has felt a total of 10 fetal movements. A significant decrease in fetal activity demands further evaluation.

Nonstress Test

The nonstress test (NST) is an ideal screening technique that is easily performed in an outpatient setting and usually requires no more than 20 minutes. The fetal heart rate is recorded with an external heart rate monitor. A normal response is the presence of two or more accelerations of at least 15 beats per minute and lasting at least 15 seconds during 20 minutes of observation. This "reactive" test is considered a reassuring finding. In a metabolically stable patient, a reactive NST will predict fetal survival for up to 1 week.

The NST may be performed weekly after 28 weeks gestation and then twice weekly at 32 weeks gestation. Because normal fetal activity and a reactive NST are rarely associated with an intrauterine fetal death, the primary value of surveillance has been to allow the clinician to delay delivery safely while the fetus gains further maturity. However, because the screening tests have significant false-positive rates, an abnormal test, e.g., as a decrease in fetal activity, must be further evaluated.

Contraction Stress Test

The contraction stress test (CST), in which uterine contractions are induced and the response of the fetal heart rate to the contractions is observed, may be required if the NST is nonreactive or suggests fetal compromise.

Biophysical Profile

Recently, some clinicians have turned to the biophysical profile to assess fetal condition. The biophysical profile utilizes real-time ultrasound to observe fetal activity, fetal breathing movements, amniotic fluid volume, and fetal tone. Like the NST, the biophysical profile can usually be completed within 15 minutes and, if normal, indicates fetal well-being.

Assessment of Fetal Growth

Fetal growth should be assessed with serial ultrasound examinations every 4 to 6 weeks to detect hydramnios and macrosomia in poorly controlled patients and growth retardation in pregnancies complicated by vasculopathy. Delivery by cesarean section should be considered if the ultrasound studies suggest excessive fetal size.

The techniques utilized today for antepartum fetal surveillance permit most patients to remain outside the hospital even during the final 4 to 6 weeks of gestation, as long as maternal control is acceptable and fetal evaluation is reassuring. Nevertheless, hospitalization may be necessary if the patient has nephropathy and/or hypertension, if she has not adhered to the regimen, or when fetal jeopardy is suspected.

TIMING OF DELIVERY

In the past, preterm delivery was often elected to avoid the risk of intrauterine fetal death. In many instances, such infants, although born alive, succumbed to respiratory distress syndrome (RDS). An increased incidence of RDS due to the combined effects of prematurity and diabetes, which may retard normal maturation of pulmonary surfactant production, was observed in infants of diabetic mothers.

Today, delivery can be safely delayed until term in most pregnancies complicated by type I diabetes. Labor may then be induced when the cervix is favorable, or the onset of spontaneous labor may be awaited. Patients must continue excellent glycemic control, and all parameters of antepartum fetal surveillance should remain normal.

In women who have vasculopathy, who have been in poor control, who have had a prior stillbirth, or who have not adhered to the program of care, elective delivery to prevent a late fetal death may be planned at 38 weeks gestation provided that fetal pulmonary maturation has been confirmed by the analysis of amniotic fluid for surfactant. RDS is highly unlikely when the amniotic fluid lecithin-to-sphingomyelin (L/S) ratio is greater than or equal to 2.0 and the acidic phospholipid phosphatidylglycerol (PG) is present.

If the fetal lungs are still immature at 38 weeks, delivery may be postponed as long as the results of fetal assessment remain reassuring. In such cases, amniocentesis should be repeated in approximately 1 week. It is essential that the obstetrician know the reliability of the analytical technique used for phospholipid analysis in the reporting laboratory, particularly in pregnancies complicated by diabetes mellitus.

Delivery despite fetal lung immaturity may be necessitated when testing suggests fetal compromise or if the pregnant patient develops preeclampsia, rapidly worsening retinopathy, or renal failure.

LABOR AND DELIVERY

The timing and site of delivery must be discussed and coordinated with the neonatologists who are to be present. If delivery is anticipated and adequate maternal or neonatal care cannot be provided, the patient should be transferred to a hospital with an appropriately equipped nursery. Expert care is required to deal with the various complications that may arise in the infant of the diabetic mother.

Intrapartum electronic monitoring of the fetal heart rate is mandatory. Labor should be allowed to progress as long as cervical dilation and descent follow the established curves for normal labor. Any evidence of an arrest pattern should alert the physician to the possibility of cephalopelvic disproportion and fetal macrosomia. An attempted vaginal delivery in this setting may lead to shoulder dystocia and birth trauma.

Maternal Glucose Levels During Delivery

Maintenance of normal maternal glucose levels (60–100 mg/dl) during labor and delivery will reduce the risk of subsequent neonatal hypoglycemia. During active labor in most patients, regardless of their antepartum insulin requirements, an intravenous solution containing 10 units of short-acting insulin in 1000 milliliters of 5% dextrose infused at 100 milliliters per hour will result in glucose levels below 100 mg/dl. Glucose levels should be determined hourly with SMBG techniques at the bedside because this dose of insulin may produce hypoglycemia during active labor. Adjustments in the delivery of insulin and/or glucose should be made based on the glucose determinations.

If labor is electively induced or a cesarean section is planned, the procedure should be scheduled for the early morning, and the patient's usual morning insulin dose should be withheld. Epidural anesthesia is preferred in patients scheduled for cesarean section. After the operation has been completed, glucose levels should be monitored every 1 to 2 hours, and an intravenous solution containing 5% dextrose should be continued. Because hPL and its contrainsulin actions fall rapidly after removal of the placenta, no insulin may be required for the remainder of the day.

POSTPARTUM CARE

In the immediate postpartum period, the patient's insulin requirements are usually lower than her prepregnancy needs. The antepartum objective of physiologic glycemic control is usually relaxed at this time. Breast-feeding is encouraged. The meal plan for the breast-feeding mother should be increased by approximately 500 calories (see **Nutrition**).

If the patient delivered vaginally, and if glucose levels are 200 mg/dl or higher, short-acting insulin may be administered as necessary on the 1st and 2nd postpartum days. On days 3 and 4, insulin dosage is based on the total insulin needed on days 1 and 2; the patient should be given two-thirds of this total dose as intermediate-acting insulin, supplemented by short-acting insulin as determined by SMBG.

In patients who have undergone a cesarean section, no insulin may be required for the first 2 or 3 postoperative days because calorie intake is limited. On days 3 and 4, short-acting insulin may be administered for glucose levels of 200 mg/dl or higher, and the following day, two-thirds of the daily total administered as intermediate-acting insulin supplemented by short-acting insulin as indicated by SMBG. Adjustment of insulin needs in the postpartum period should always be individualized based on SMBG results.

FAMILY PLANNING AND CONTRACEPTION

Family planning and contraception must be reviewed with the patient during the postpartum period. Although oral contraceptives are the most effective method available, the increased risk of thromboembolic disease and vasculopathy require that combined estrogen/progestin oral-contraceptive preparations be used with caution; only low-dose estrogen agents should be prescribed. Combination agents are contraindicated in women with hypertension or vasculopathy, who may be offered a progestin-only pill instead.

Motivated patients may do well with a barrier method of contraception such as the diaphragm, although their efficacy is significantly lower than that of oral contraceptives. Sterilization should be discussed with the patient when she has completed her family or if she has serious vasculopathy.

CONCLUSION

Advances in biochemical and electronic monitoring techniques have markedly improved maternal and fetal well-being in pregnancy complicated by diabetes. Meticulous metabolic control before and during pregnancy holds the key to a successful outcome and to minimizing fetal malformations or neonatal complications. A team approach is more likely to achieve a desirable result.

BIBLIOGRAPHY

Cohen AW, Gabbe SG: Intrapartum management of the diabetic patient. Cl. *Perinatology* 8:165–72, 1981

Freinkel N: Banting Lecture 1980: of pregnancy and progeny. *Diabetes* 29:1023–35, 1980

Fuhrmann K, Reiher H, Semmler K, Fischer F, Fischer M, Glöckner E: Prevention of congenital malformations in infants of insulin-dependent diabetic mothers. *Diabetes Care* 6:219–23, 1983

Gabbe SG: Management of diabetes mellitus in pregnancy. *Am J Obstet Gynecol* 153:824–28, 1985

Jovanovic L, Fuhrmann K, Peterson CM: *Diabetes in Pregnancy: Teratology, Toxicology, and Treatment.* New York, Praeger, 1985

Steel JM, Johnstone FD, Smith AF, Duncan LJP: Five years experience of "prepregnancy" clinic for insulin-dependent diabetes. *Br Med J* 285: 353–56, 1982

Surgery

INTRODUCTION

The physician caring for patients with insulin-dependent (type I) diabetes mellitus should become familiar with proper pre- and postoperative management during elective or emergency surgery. It is now possible for a patient with diabetes to undergo surgery with little more than normal risk, given sufficient time for complete patient evaluation and preparation. Guidelines for diabetes management during both elective and emergency surgery are presented herein.

GENERAL PRINCIPLES

The objectives of glycemic management before, during, and after an operation are to prevent hypoglycemia as well as excessive hyperglycemia and ketoacidosis. Insulin requirements often increase during the acute stress of a major surgical procedure, despite the fact that the patient may not be eating. For this reason, the patient's customary basal insulin dosage is usually continued throughout the perioperative period. Supplemental insulin may also be needed to prevent excessive hepatic glucose release and resulting hyperglycemia. Normal fluid and electrolyte balance should be maintained, and oral feedings should be resumed as soon as possible.

Although ideally the plasma glucose level should be kept near that of nondiabetic individuals at all times, precision of control is difficult to achieve in practice and increases the risk of hypoglycemia; therefore, it is generally considered safer to err on the side of mild hyperglycemia. Although some evidence suggests that perioperative hyperglycemia may delay healing, the risks are small compared with those of hypoglycemia in a patient whose mental status is already altered by anesthesia or postoperative medications.

Plasma glucose levels between 150 and 250 mg/dl during and after the operation are considered to be satisfactory. With a highly skilled operative/postoperative team and readily available monitoring, blood glucose may be targeted to remain between 120 and 180 mg/dl.

Medical management of the patient with diabetes will depend on whether the surgery is emergency or elective and whether the anesthesia to be used is general or local.

GENERAL ANESTHESIA

Elective Surgery

The patient scheduled for elective surgery should be allowed sufficient time to achieve the best possible general health and control of blood glucose before admission to the hospital. Complete evaluation of metabolic state and thorough assessment of diabetic complications, including renal and heart disease, is highly desirable before surgery.

The primary-care physician, surgeon, and anesthesiologist (preferably one experienced in diabetes management during surgery) should cooperate in preparing the diabetic patient for surgery. The anesthetic technique chosen should minimize disruption of metabolic control, and if possible, the operation should be scheduled for early morning to avoid prolonged fasting. This also makes it more likely that any postoperative metabolic care can be suitably provided.

In the past few years, an increasing number of authorities have advocated intravenous infusion of insulin rather than subcutaneous administration during the perioperative period. Intravenous infusion allows careful control of the amount and speed of insulin delivery and circumvents problems in the event of peripheral shutdown (e.g., hypotension, shock), which might occur during major surgery. For these reasons, *intravenous insulin delivery is preferred during surgery.*

Suggested guidelines for management of diabetic patients by use of intravenous insulin can be found in Box 26. Guidelines for the subcutaneous route are in Box 27.

Emergency Surgery

In the event of emergency surgery requiring general anesthesia, there may

Box 26. Intravenous Insulin Regimen for Elective Surgery

Preoperative Days

Attempt to obtain reasonable glycemic control (i.e., preprandial glucose concentrations >80 mg/dl but <180 mg/dl). If necessary, admit patient 2–3 days before surgery for this purpose. Most patients will require at least 2 injections of intermediate-acting insulin; many will require additional preprandial short-acting insulin. Insulin-dose adjustments are generally based on preprandial glucose concentrations at 0800, 1200, 1800, and 2200 h.

Operative Day

On the morning of surgery, keep patient NPO, omit usual subcutaneous insulin, and insert intravenous infusion line.

Start infusion of 5 g/h dextrose (D5W or D10W) with 2 meq/h KCl.

Administer insulin as follows.

- Begin with infusion of 1 U/h short-acting insulin.
- Evaluate blood glucose with reflectance meter every 4 h before surgery, *every hour* during surgery, and every 4 h after surgery.
- Do not change infusion rate if blood glucose remains between 120 and 180 mg/dl.
- Increase infusion rate by 0.5 U/h if blood glucose value is >180 mg/dl.
- Decrease infusion rate by 0.5 U/h if blood glucose value is <120 mg/dl.

NOTE: In children, the hourly rate of fluid infusion is adjusted to be consistent with daily maintenance fluid requirements of ~1500 ml/m^2 body surface area. Nevertheless, 1 U insulin/5 g glucose should be infused.

After Surgery

When meals are resumed, discontinue intravenous insulin infusion and resume subcutaneous insulin as described in Box 27.

The simplicity of this regimen and the ease of adjustment of insulin or glucose infusion rates have made it the preferred mode of insulin delivery during surgery.

not be sufficient time to optimally evaluate and stabilize the patient. Patients with diabetic ketoacidosis (DKA) who need emergency surgery represent a particular problem. In these patients, efforts should be made to delay surgery until the ketoacidosis is treated, even if not to complete resolution (as described in **Ketoacidosis**).

If surgery cannot be postponed, treatment of DKA should be initiated (as described in **Ketoacidosis,** p. 63) and continued throughout the operative and perioperative period. Once blood glucose has fallen below 300 mg/dl, insulin should be continued but at the rate described in Box 26.

Potassium should be checked frequently (every 1–2 h for the first 4 h and every 3–4 h thereafter). If potassium is normal or low with acidosis, intravenous potassium should be started at a rate of 10 to 15 meq/h and the rate adjusted according to plasma concentration determined at the intervals above. These guidelines are similar to those described in **Ketoacidosis.**

LOCAL ANESTHESIA

Patients undergoing elective surgery with local anesthesia (e.g., dental work) generally should eat only after surgery, and surgery should preferably be scheduled as the first case to minimize duration of fasting. Insulin dose should be decreased on the morning of surgery. One approach is to give half of the customary dose of intermediate-acting insulin or the full dose of long-acting insulin. Short-acting insulin should be omitted.

Glucose concentrations should be measured before surgery. If glucose exceeds 240 mg/dl by color estimation or 300 mg/dl by meter, a small amount of short-acting insulin should be given with an algorithm similar to that given in Box 27.

If glucose is less than 60 mg/dl postoperatively, an intravenous bolus of glucose (~1 g for each 5- to 10-mg/dl increment in blood glucose desired) should be given or the patient allowed to eat or drink. Generally, the custom-

Box 27. Subcutaneous Insulin Regimen for Elective Surgery

Preoperative Days

See Box 26.

Operative Day

On the morning of surgery, keep patient NPO and adjust dose in the following manner (patient's basal insulin requirements continue during the perioperative period).

Usual Type of Insulin	Morning of Surgery
Intermediate acting	50% of usual dose
Short acting	Omit
Long acting (e.g., ultralente)	Usual dose
Continuous subcutaneous insulin infusion	Usual basal coverage

Start an intravenous infusion of dextrose (D5W). In adults, set rate at ~100 ml/h. In children, the hourly rate is adjusted to be consistent with daily fluid requirements of ~1500 ml/m² body surface area.

During Surgery

Insulin. Inject small amounts of subcutaneous insulin if glucose is >200 mg/dl, according to the suggested algorithm below. In prepubertal children, halve these amounts.

Glucose (mg/dl)	Insulin (U)
200–250	2–4
250–300	4–6
≥300	6–8

Give supplemental subcutaneous insulin only every 4 h. Decrease glucose infusion rate if blood glucose concentration continues to rise.

Glucose. Continue infusion of dextrose (D5W) at a rate of ~100 ml/h, or as appropriate for children.

The following are regimens for treating low blood glucose.

- If ≤80 mg/dl, increase glucose infusion rate by 50%.
- If ≤60 mg/dl or
- if patient is symptomatic, give an intravenous bolus of glucose (~1 g per 5- to 10-mg/dl increment in blood glucose desired); if fluid volume is a consideration, D10W or D20W may be used rather than D5W.

After Surgery

Insulin-Glucose Regimen. Continue subcutaneous supplements and dextrose (D5W) infusion until oral feeding is resumed.

If patient is NPO for several days, infuse sufficient glucose (150–200 g/day in adults; 2–4 $g \cdot kg^{-1} \cdot day^{-1}$ in children) to meet minimal catabolic needs.

Adjust the insulin infusion [initially ~10 U/L dextrose (D5W)] to prevent hyperglycemia or hypoglycemia.

Transition to Oral Feeding. If patient is able to eat and on a program that includes

- *preprandial short-acting insulin plus evening intermediate-acting insulin*: 30 min before a meal, inject sufficient short-acting insulin to cover ingested calories. If necessary, supplement with short-acting insulin according to the above algorithm. The meal should be available at the nursing station before the patient receives insulin. Give late-evening dose of immediate-acting insulin as usual.
- *intermediate-acting insulin* only: modify evening dose of intermediate-acting insulin in proportion to the number of calories consumed during the day.
- *long-acting or continuous subcutaneous insulin infusion*: continue customary basal dose of long-acting insulin or the basal rate of insulin infusion pump.

In all cases, monitor blood glucose every 4 h. Give supplements of insulin or glucose depending on self-monitoring of blood glucose results. When meals are fully tolerated, the presurgery insulin regimen can be reinstituted.

Succeeding Postoperative Days

Insulin dose will rise as the patient's calorie intake increases. Blood glucose measured before meals and at bedtime should be used to guide insulin dose adjustments.

ary meal plan and insulin program may be continued postoperatively. This may require supplemental blood glucose monitoring with adjustments of insulin based on premeal blood glucose levels.

In the case of emergency surgery requiring a local anesthesia, every effort should be made to measure blood glucose concentration before surgery begins; the guidelines above should be followed.

CONCLUSION

Medical management of the diabetic patient requiring surgery must focus on provision of glucose and insulin in amounts to avoid hypoglycemia or hyperglycemia during and after surgery. Intravenous insulin and glucose at a rate providing approximately 1 unit of short-acting insulin for each 5 grams of glucose and frequent blood glucose monitoring will usually keep blood glucose levels between 120 and 250 mg/dl. Major elective surgery in a diabetic patient is best performed in centers capable of integrating anesthetic, surgical, and medical care in a team approach.

BIBLIOGRAPHY

Husband DJ, Thai AC, Alberti KGMM: Management of diabetes during surgery with glucose-insulin-potassium infusion. *Diabetic Med* 3: 69–74, 1986

Johnston DG, Alberti KGMM: Diabetic emergencies: practical aspects of the management of diabetic ketoacidosis and diabetes during surgery. *Clin Endocrinol Metab* 9:437–60, 1980

Meyer EJ, Lorenzi M, Bohannon NV, Amend W, Fedeska NJ, Salvatierra O, Forsham TH: Diabetic management by insulin infusion during major surgery. *Am J Surg* 137:323–27, 1979

Pezzarossa A, Taddei F, Cimicchi MC, Rossini E, Contini S, Bonoro E, Gnudi A, Uggeri E: Perioperative management of diabetic subjects: subcutaneous versus intravenous insulin administration during glucose-potassium infusion. *Diabetes Care* 11: 52–58, 1988

Walts LF, Miller J, Davidson MB, Brown J: Perioperative management of diabetes mellitus. *Anesthesiology* 55:104–109, 1981

Psychosocial Problems: Helping Patients Cope

Highlights
Psychosocial Problems: Helping Patients Cope

COPING WITH DIABETES

At diagnosis, emotional reactions may include shock, denial, negotiation, and anger. By providing emotional support and appropriate information, the physician can help the patient through this period successfully.

Over many years of diabetes, motivation to maintain optimal diabetes control may wane. A chief task is creating a workable diabetes regimen and helping the patient adhere to it.

When chronic complications begin, feelings of anger and guilt are common. These emotional reactions must be resolved before normal psychosocial functioning can resume.

Age-specific concerns are covered on page 93.

The physician should relate to the patient in a consultive rather than directive manner. Advantages of this approach include the following.

- It makes the treatment plan realistic to the patient's circumstances.
- It encourages the patient to seek information about problems instead of concealing failure.
- It improves adherence to difficult treatment regimens.

Common causes of nonadherence include

- lack of practical knowledge;
- lack of sense of vulnerability, control, and benefit;
- occupational, social, and familial barriers to adherence; and
- fear of hypoglycemia.

Psychological stress may interact with blood glucose control in various ways (p. 95). Before responding to patient complaints that stress is affecting blood glucose control, the physician must clarify which interaction is occurring.

Both psychogenic and organic impotence are common among diabetic men. Information in Table 18 (p. 96) can help to distinguish between the two. Other behavioral issues are discussed on page 96.

SPECIAL PROBLEMS: THE ADOLESCENT

Almost all adolescents display behaviors that reflect their drive for independence. Although these sometimes upset the diabetes regimen, **major difficulties are not inevitable.** Adolescents with diabetes suffer from serious psychological problems no more frequently than their nondiabetic peers.

Many factors other than the diabetes regimen may be critical to management. Factors known to influence adherence by adolescent patients fall into four major categories.

- **The clinic** (p. 98): convenience, waiting time, use of appointment reminders, and respect shown to adolescent
- **The patient** (p. 99): staff understanding of patient interest and abilities allows establishment of dialogue and clearly written instructions
- **The physician and health-care team** (p. 99): genuineness of physician interest in teen, development of nonparental relationship with teen, physician confidence in diabetes management ability, willingness to compromise, and caretaker consistency
- **The regimen** (p. 100): simplicity, well-documented negotiations, and short-term compromise for long-term success

Other common problems and issues include alcohol and drugs, sexual activity and contraception, driving privileges, participation in sports, misrepresenting facts, recurrent DKA, progress toward independent management of diabetes, and support groups and camps (p. 100–102).

SPECIAL PROBLEMS: THE AGED

In older insulin-requiring patients, maintaining function and general well-being should take precedence over striving for glycemic targets. The diabetes treatment regimen should be kept simple and should focus on avoiding hypoglycemia and symptomatic hyperglycemia.

For the new insulin user, the regimen should entail the fewest restrictions and changes in life routine. Nutrition goals should be kept modest. The meal plan should be balanced, consistent, and as much in concert with long-standing eating habits as possible.

One daily blood glucose measurement taken before breakfast is usually adequate, supplemented by regular glycosylated hemoglobin tests to assess overall glycemic control.

Both diabetes complications and other sources of disability should be aggressively sought and treated (p. 104–105). Of special importance are

- retinopathy,
- foot examination at every clinic visit,
- blood pressure,
- mental status, and
- reading acuity and hearing.

Maintaining the ability to walk and to see can mean the difference between independent living at home and institutionalization.

Individualization is of utmost importance—age in years is not synonymous with aging or loss of vigor.

Coping With Diabetes

INTRODUCTION

Although insulin-dependent (type I) diabetes taxes the patient's psychosocial well-being, the converse is also true: psychosocial factors affect diabetes management. The unrelenting demands of treatment and the threat of early disability or death put tremendous strain on the diabetic patient and the family. The patient will simultaneously be attempting to manage the more usual personal and age-specific concerns of life. In helping the patient cope with diabetes, the physician must consider the evolving disease, the developmental stage of the patient, and the interaction between the two.

THE EVOLVING DISEASE

From a psychosocial perspective, diabetes can be considered to develop in three phases: diagnosis, maintenance, and later chronic complications.

Diagnosis Phase

The weeks or months after diagnosis require emotional adjustment for both patient and family (Box 28). Typically, this process follows the five stages of classic grieving. They include initial shock, denial, negotiation, anger, and acceptance.

During the diagnosis phase, the patient and family should be given only the most basic medical information. Most individuals cannot absorb new knowledge readily, whereas others will focus exclusively on the facts, denying the emotional impact of the disease. The physician can be of great help during this period by being accessible and sensitive to the patient's need to have information repeated several times. Eventually, when patients are ready to go beyond the fundamentals, it may be helpful for them to meet other families (from the physician's practice or local diabetes groups) who are also dealing with diabetes.

It is important that the whole family accept the reality of life with diabetes and the realistic restrictions it imposes. Psychotherapy may be helpful if the resolution of the diagnosis phase is not completed within 1 year.

Box 28. Factors Causing Emotional Distress at Diagnosis

Agents of stress include the following.

- Uncertainty about the outcome of the immediate situation
- Feelings of intense guilt and/or anger about the occurrence of diabetes
- Feelings of incompetence and helplessness about the responsibility for management of the illness
- Fears about future complications and early death
- Loss of valued life goals and aspirations because of illness
- Anxiety about planning for an uncertain future
- Recognition of the necessity for a permanent change in living pattern due to diabetes

Adapted from Hamburg BA, Inoff GE: Coping with predictable crises of diabetes. *Diabetes Care* 6:409–16, 1983

Maintenance Phase

The maintenance phase begins once the patient and family have learned to live with the disease and extends until the onset of chronic complications. Motivation to maintain optimal control can wane on the part of the patient, the family, and the physician. A chief task of the lengthy maintenance period is creating a workable diabetes regimen and helping the patient adhere to it.

Complication Phase

This phase is associated with development of complications such as retinopathy, circulatory difficulties, and renal failure. Once again, the patient must grieve, this time over blindness, amputation, dialysis, or impotence. Feelings of anger at the physician for "letting it happen" or guilt ("I should have taken better care of myself") are common. The multiple emotional reactions that characterize the complication phase must be resolved before normal psychosocial functioning can resume.

Table 15. Impact of Diagnosis

	PARENTS	CHILD
Infant	Shock, disbelief, denial, anger, guilt, depression. Affects capacity to learn regimen.	Responds to added tension and discomfort.
Toddler	Shock, disbelief, denial, anger, guilt, depression. Affects capacity to learn regimen.	Regression: motor, speech development, toilet training.
Preschool	Shock, disbelief, denial, anger, guilt, depression. Affects capacity to learn regimen.	Regression in social behavior and skills. May "cling" more.
School age	Shock, disbelief, denial, anger, guilt, depression. Affects capacity to learn regimen.	Depression, regression; withdrawal from social, athletic activities; school work may be affected. Aware of genetic factors.
Adolescence	Shock, disbelief, denial, anger, guilt, depression. Affects capacity to learn regimen.	Similar to adult grieving; recognizes implication of diabetes, potential complications. Aware of genetic factors.
Young adult	Shock, disbelief, denial, anger, guilt, depression. Affects capacity to learn regimen.	Similar to adult grieving; recognizes implication of diabetes, potential complications. Aware of genetic factors.

DKA, diabetic ketoacidosis.

THE CHANGING PATIENT

Children

Generally, children's responsibilities for care should increase in tandem with cognitive and psychological development (Tables 15–17). Active participation is important because the more ownership the child has in treatment, the better adherence and control can be. When treating the school-age child, the physician should be alert to cognitive deficits that may interfere with drawing the correct amount of insulin, accurately interpreting self-monitoring of blood glucose (SMBG) results, or calculating the number of calories consumed.

Family tensions may revolve around the diabetic member: a healthy sibling may feel neglected. Marital conflict and even child abuse sometimes occur. For these reasons, the diabetic child is best treated as part of a family unit, which the physician should monitor closely and intervene in if necessary.

The health-care team should ensure that school personnel are aware of the child's diabetes and are knowledgeable about coping with insulin reactions, the effect of hypoglycemia on behavior and thinking, and whom to call in case of an emergency. Ideally, school personnel should also be familiar with SMBG.

Adolescents

Striking hormonal changes during puberty and increased emphasis on autonomy and peer pressure can make a previously cooperative child become overtly (or covertly) rebellious. In its spontaneity, particularly with regard to eating and activity, typical adolescent behavior directly conflicts with the treatment regimen, and often adolescents will conform to peer-group norms rather than to those of parents or physicians.

Deliberate manipulation of the diabetes regimen for personal ends, e.g., underinsulinizing to lose weight, is common. Alternatively, diabetes may be used to cope with the issues of adolescence. Excuses about the need for dietary adherence may be invoked to avoid social encounters; self-induced insulin reactions or even diabetic ketoacidosis (DKA) may be engineered as a way around social or family conflicts. Smoking, substance abuse, and sex should be discussed in a frank and straightforward manner.

Adults

Marriage and family, employment, finances, and anticipation of complications are some of the chief concerns of adulthood. When entering into marriage, the patient's spouse must learn what diabetes is, how to manage common crises, and how to support adherence to the treatment regimen. Some discussion of long-term complications is appropriate. Both partners should understand the risks of pregnancy for the diabetic woman and the need for glycemia to be optimal at the time of conception to minimize the risk of congenital malformations (see **Pregnancy**).

Physician and patient should work together to match the regimen to the realities of the patient's job (e.g., shift work, frequent restaurant meals, or special eating or physical activity patterns). Patients who operate machinery or heavy equipment should be cautioned about the danger of even mild hypoglycemia on the job.

The special needs of elderly patients are discussed in **The Aged.**

DOCTOR-PATIENT RELATIONSHIP

Because the patient with diabetes has the responsibility for routine treatment, a visit to the physician usually involves consultation about the regimen instead of direct provision of treatment. Giving advice and reaching mutual agreements should constitute a major part of each office visit.

A "consultative" approach has several advantages. It

- makes the treatment plan realistic for the patient's circumstances,
- encourages the patient to seek information during difficult diabetes management (instead of avoiding the physician or distorting information about treatment failure), and
- improves adherence to difficult treatment regimens.

The physician should guard against unrealistically high expectations and be flexible enough to compromise the ideal treatment plan. It is essential to praise the patient for whatever treatment successes are achieved, rather than to criticize perceived failures. Such a realistic supportive approach lays the groundwork for future collaboration and progressive improvement of the treatment plan.

Research has shown that most patients forget 50% of what was said immediately after leaving the doctor's office. Therefore, it is important to write down any "behavioral prescriptions," perhaps even on a prescription pad. This

Table 16. Major Development Issues

Infant	Trusting relationship: interaction with parents about food.
Toddler	Early steps toward autonomy: balkiness, stubbornness. Exploration of environment without judgment.
Preschool	Intense concerns about body strength and "intactness." May view diabetes management as "punishment." Fears injections and blood testing as bodily injury.
School age	Curiosity, development of motor, intellectual, social skills. Attachment shifts gradually from family to peers: sensitive to feeling "adequate."
Adolescence	Identity formation, intense body awareness, sexual identity. Dependence-independence struggle with parents and authorities: defiance. Measures self against peers; diabetes may make feel less adequate.
Young adult	Emotional ties to family lessen; career development; interpersonal commitment. Concerns about possible diabetes complications and effect on future goals.

Table 17. Management Implications

	PARENTS	PROFESSIONALS
Infant	Difficulties in differentiating hypoglycemic reactions from 'normal'' distress. Monitoring of diabetes felt as "overwhelming" and "lonely."	Constant availability of medical team.
Toddler	Temper tantrums in child interfere with distinguishing insulin reactions, giving injections, and blood tests.	Select least painful sites for injections and blood tests.
Preschool	Normal moodiness easily confused with hypoglycemic reactions.	Select least painful sites for injections and blood tests.
School age	Encourage self-monitoring: recognize hypoglycemic reactions; participate in diet planning; help in blood testing; draw up and occasionally inject insulin. *All activities to be supervised.*	Begin seeing child alone during office visits.
Adolescence	Experimentation: omitting insulin and blood testing, not following diet; in extreme situations DKA and recurrent DKA indicates need for psychiatric intervention. Discretion needed in physical contact: information about sexuality and diabetes beneficial. Capable of some self-management, still needing overall adult supervision and involvement.	As "neutral" adult assure confidentiality and privacy at visits.
Young adult	*Young adult* responsible for diabetes management; shares information with others.	Continuing relationship beneficial to prepare for possible future physical complications.

DKA, diabetic ketoacidosis.

can help facilitate both recall and adherence.

FACILITATING ADHERENCE

There are several factors to consider in facilitating adherence (see **Education**), i.e.,

- practical knowledge;
- sense of vulnerability, control, and benefit;
- occupational, social, and familial barriers to adherence; and
- fear of hypoglycemia.

The degree to which patients are willing to participate in their treatment will be influenced by their perception of *vulnerability* to the complications of diabetes, sense of control over their disease, or the perceived benefits of aherence to delaying and/or preventing the long-term complications of diabetes.

Even if knowledgeable and cooperative, a patient may confront significant barriers to appropriate self-care. Food preferences of other family members may undermine the prescribed meal plan, and simple difficulties with transportation may make appropriate food or medicine hard to obtain. Adherence may be impeded by an unsupportive spouse, parent, teacher, or boss.

Fear of hypoglycemia is common among diabetic patients. Because hypoglycemic episodes can be both embarassing and frightening, patients (or their parents) may attempt to avert insulin reactions by keeping blood glucose inappropriately high as a safety margin.

There are several excellent articles covering the subject of adherence (see Bibliography).

ESTIMATING BLOOD GLUCOSE LEVELS

Many patients who use SMBG do so only infrequently because they do not know how to use the information obtained or because of the expense, pain, and inconvenience involved.

Instead, many patients estimate blood glucose level by "feel." In fact, patients experienced with SMBG are reasonably accurate at estimating glycemic extremes on the basis of symptoms. When they think they are either hypo- or hyperglycemic, they are frequently correct. Consequently, mature patients should be encouraged to treat themselves if they feel hypoglycemic. Monitoring of blood glucose should be performed for younger children.

The most common patient error in blood glucose estimation is believing that blood glucose is normal when in fact it is either too high or too low. For this reason, patients should be encouraged to measure their blood glucose at times when they feel it is normal.

STRESS AND BLOOD GLUCOSE LEVELS

Patients commonly complain of the disruptive effects of stress (usually referring to psychological stress) on their diabetes. Because psychological stress and glycemic control interact in several ways, this broad statement must be clarified before action is taken (Figure 4).

Figure 4. Interactions Between Psychological Stress and Glycemic Control

	Direct	Indirect
Stress → Blood glucose	Stress hormones	Disrupt adherence
Blood glucose → Stress	Misinterpret adrenergic symptoms	Disruptive neuroglycopenic symptoms

- Psychological stress can affect metabolic control *directly* by stimulating the release of blood glucose–raising hormones like epinephrine. Less commonly, stressed individuals experience decreases in blood glucose because they omit food.
- Symptoms of stress may be confused with those of hypoglycemia. Patients may misinterpret the adrenergic symptoms of hypoglycemia (palpitations and sweating) as psychological stress.
- Stress may also *indirectly* influence diabetes control by disrupting the treatment regimen. Patients under stress may forget to take their insulin on time, measure the dose incorrectly, eat too much or too little, and exercise more or less than usual.
- Finally, neuroglycopenic symptoms of severe hypoglycemia can disrupt work or social functioning, leading to compromising and embarrassing situations and, thus, indirectly causing stress.

Evaluating Stress

When patients complain that stress is interfering with diabetes control, the physician must clarify whether the patient is talking about the direct effects on blood glucose or the indirect effects on adherence. In the case of the former, the next step is to determine whether the patient is experiencing psychological stress or the adrenergic effects of hypoglycemia; this can be accomplished by monitoring blood glucose whenever such symptoms occur. If stress is found to be affecting metabolic control directly, behavioral or pharmacological stress-management intervention may be indicated.

SEXUALITY

Physician and patient may be hesitant to broach the issue of sexual dysfunction. However, sexuality is an important component of self-esteem and marital functioning. If sexuality is not spontaneously discussed by the patient, it is critical that the physician bring up the topic in a frank straightforward manner. When sexual difficulties are not resolved after open discussion and possible use of written and audiovisual materials, referral to psychotherapy may be considered.

Sexual Dysfunction in Men

Both psychogenic and organic impotence are common among diabetic men. Use of *The Male Sexual Functioning Questionnaire* can help to distinguish between the two (Table 18). If the patient answers "true" to three or fewer of these questions, impotence is probably psychogenic, and sexual counseling should be considered. If four or more answers are true, then the impotence could be either psychogenic or organic, and nocturnal tumescence studies are indicated. A simple first step is the "postage-stamp" test, in which the patient places a ring of postage stamps around the flaccid penis at bedtime; if the band of stamps is not broken during sleep, organic impotence may be suspected, and the patient should be referred to a urologist for further investigation and treatment.

Table 18. Male Sexual Functioning Questionnaire

T F	Every time I try to get an erection it is less than 100% full.
T F	I never wake up in the morning or during the night with a 100% full erection.
T F	It frequently or always takes me longer to reach ejaculation than it used to.
T F	During oral sex or masturbation, I always get less than 100% full erection.
T F	The amount I ejaculate is frequently or always less than it used to be.
T F	I rarely or never ejaculate prematurely (too soon).
T F	I frequently or always fail to get a 100% full erection.

Psychogenic, fewer than 4 clear "T" responses.

Adapted from Abel GG, Becker JV, Cunningham-Rathner J, Mittelman M, Primack M: Differential diagnosis of impotence in diabetics: the validity of sexual symptomatology. *Neurourol Urodyn* 1:57–69, 1982

Options for management of organic impotence include
- no treatment,
- sexual counseling to develop alternative forms of mutual sexual gratification, or
- penile prostheses, often supplemented by sex therapy to aid in adjustment, see also **Neuropathy,** p. 128.

Sexual Dysfunction in Women

Some data indicate that women with long-standing diabetes lose the ability to lubricate during sexual arousal and experience a general loss of libido. Lubricant preparations are readily available without a prescription. Loss of libido is best dealt with by counseling the couple.

OTHER BEHAVIORAL ISSUES

Alcohol. High blood alcohol levels can interfere with the body's ability to counterregulate. Intoxication can also interfere with adherence to self-management regimens. For this reason, alcohol abuse should always be considered in nonadherent adults.

Smoking. Patients should be asked directly if they smoke, preferably when the spouse is present, and advised of the special dangers smoking presents to people with diabetes. For some patients, being told that smoking increases the possibility of amputations or death is sufficient to prompt quitting. Others who are interested in quitting but who have some difficulty may be referred to a smoking cessation program.

Eating Disorders. Bulimia is an increasing problem, especially among young adult women. Because this behavior is not always obvious during a patient's visit, and because it can play havoc with metabolic control, the physician should always inquire about "binging and purging" with late adolescent and young adult females (Box 29). If the condition is present or even suspected, a referral should be made to a psychologist or psychiatrist specializing in this condition.

CONCLUSION

Because of the evolving nature of the patient and the disease, there are always new challenges for the patient, family, and physician. The issues of diabetes management, if handled appropriately, can actually enhance a patient's ability to deal with other life crises.

Box 29. Red Flags for Possible Bulimia

The following signs could indicate bulimia.

- Excessive concern about weight
- Strict dieting followed by eating binges
- Frequent overeating, especially when distressed
- Binging on high-caloric sweet food
- Expressing guilt or shame about eating
- Being secretive about binges and vomiting
- Feeling out of control
- Disappearing after meals
- Depressed mood
- Rapid weight fluctuations within a normal weight range
- Frequent use of purging and/or laxatives

BIBLIOGRAPHY

American Diabetes Association: Techniques for helping the patient cope with diagnosis and treatment. In *The Physician's Guide to Non-Insulin-Dependent (Type II) Diabetes: Diagnosis and Treatment.* Alexandria, VA, Am. Diabetes Assoc., 1988, p. 57–64

Cerkoney KAB, Hart LK: The relationship between health belief model and compliance of persons with diabetes mellitus. *Diabetes Care* 3:594–98, 1980

Cox DJ, Gonder-Frederick LA: *Behavioral Medicine Handbook of Diabetes Mellitus.* Champagne, IL, Research Press, 1988

Eraker SA, Becker MH: Improving compliance for the patient with diabetes. *Diabetes Prof* August:22–27, 1987

Eraker SA, Kirscht JP, Becker MH: Understanding and improving patient compliance. *Ann Intern Med* 100: 258–68, 1984

Special Problems: The Adolescent

INTRODUCTION

Management of insulin-dependent (type I) diabetes mellitus during the adolescent years is notoriously difficult. For the young child with diabetes, successful adherence to the treatment regimen depends largely on parental interest and management skills. In contrast, few adolescents will accept complete parental control of their diabetes, yet most are incapable of or unwilling to fully care for themselves. Furthermore, many aspects of the care regimen are at odds with the adolescent's drive for independence and peer acceptance.

Consequently, adolescents may neglect monitoring, dietary considerations, insulin injections, and even visits to the clinic. These actions can bring disastrous consequences both in the short and long term. The clinician can use various strategies to help the adolescent patient and family keep diabetes control within acceptable limits.

SCOPE OF THE PROBLEM

Almost all adolescents display characteristic behaviors and attitudes that reflect their drive for independence. Adolescents with diabetes are no exception. They undergo the same developmental process but with the added burden of diabetes. Hence, the physician who cares for adolescents with diabetes should be prepared for a challenge.

However, the clinician need not assume that major difficulties are inevitable. There is no evidence that adolescents with diabetes suffer from serious psychological problems more frequently than their nondiabetic peers. Moreover, most adolescents, with or without diabetes, manage to navigate this sometimes stormy period without incurring any major psychological or physical repercussions.

Many hormonal changes occur at puberty, some of which can affect blood glucose levels. Puberty is associated with decreased sensitivity to insulin, and this may dictate an increase in insulin requirement. Once dose adjustments have been made, an adolescent's further problems in controlling diabetes can usually be linked to psychological rather than physical factors.

FACTORS AFFECTING ADHERENCE

Factors known to influence adherence of adolescent patients can be grouped into four major categories (Box 30):

- the clinic setting
- the patient
- the physician and other members of the health-care team
- the regimen

Clinic Setting

Clinic or office factors may affect patient adherence to the medical regimen. One important factor is convenience. Does the patient have to travel a long distance to the clinic? Are there adequate parking facilities? Is there flexibility in scheduling of appointments?

Clinic staff should be friendly and careful not to treat the adolescent as a child. They should speak directly to the patient, not just with the parents. Similarly, staff should reduce waiting time to a minimum. The adolescent may be angry at being forcibly brought to the clinic, and a long wait may increase anger to the point that the visit is unproductive.

At each visit, patients should be asked if they want their parents present during the history and/or physical examination. If the parents do not participate in the clinic visit, it is important that they be informed of the patient's progress and the physician's recommendations. However, this report should take place while the adolescent is present. Secret meetings between clinician and parents can destroy trust in the physician and threaten the adolescent's sense of independence in managing diabetes.

One of the most important predictors of adherence is the patient's success at remembering and understanding instructions. Therefore, instructions should be written and very specific. A record of the instructions permits discussion of expectations with the patient at the next clinic visit.

The Patient

Because psychosocial factors may also affect adherence, the physician should develop a psychosocial data base on each adolescent patient. This should include information about other family members and the patient's interaction with them.

Moreover, the physician should try to learn about the parent-adolescent relationship. Are there many conflicts? Does the adolescent feel burdened with too much responsibility or not entrusted with enough? What are the patient's likes and dislikes, special interests, special skills? Such information aids the physician in finding topics to discuss with the patient.

Angry adolescents may not want to discuss their diabetes at clinic visits but will often be willing to share information about some other aspect of life, e.g., a motorcycle or a volleyball tournament. Once dialogue is established, the patient usually becomes much less angry, and it is possible to address some aspect of the diabetes.

Physician's Role*

In addition to acquiring an understanding of normal adolescent development, the physician should enjoy working with adolescents and should show a genuine interest in them as individuals. If the physician cannot develop more than a superficial relationship, success in managing diabetes may not be possible. Likewise, physicians must have confidence in their diabetes management skills. If the physician is not comfortable working with adolescents or lacks the needed experience or resources, referral to a specialist should be considered.

Developing Rapport

The physician should establish rapport with the patient but must avoid becoming part of the adolescent process itself. If the physician is viewed by the adolescent negatively, as a surrogate parent, recommendations will be viewed in the same way as parental demands and may be rejected. Hence, physicians must distance themselves from the parents during interactions with adolescents.

To avoid being viewed as a parental figure, physicians should tell both the parents and the adolescent that they have responsibilities to each. At times the physician may disagree with the parents about some aspect of diabetes care and at other times disagree with the adolescent. The purpose of these discussions is to convince the adolescent that the physician-patient relationship is not one between physician and child but one between physician and young adult.

*Here, the term *physician* refers to all members of the health-care professional team, including nurse, educator, dietitian, and social worker.

Box 30. Factors That Improve Adherence

Clinic factors

- Convenient clinic location and facilities
- Flexible appointment times
- Staff sensitivity toward patient-parent interactions
- Consistent use of appointment reminders

Patient factors

- Clearly written, easily understood instructions
- Good staff understanding of patient-parent conflicts and patient interests

Physician factors

- Consistent care provided by a single physician or team

Provider requirements

- Understand diabetes management and normal adolescent development
- Enjoy working with adolescents
- Confidence in diabetes management skills
- Develop a nonparental relationship with the patient
- Willing to compromise on aspects of diabetes care

Regimen factors

- A simple regimen
- Emphasis that monitoring benefits the *patient*
- Well-documented negotiations and parent understanding of management goals
- Short-term compromise for long-term success

Willingness to Compromise

The physician must be willing to compromise on almost all aspects of diabetes care and must clearly show respect for the adolescent's views. If the physician becomes frustrated and angry when the adolescent does not adhere to the regimen, it will be difficult to influence the patient's self-care. It is not necessary to agree with the adolescent's views, but the physician should at least listen to the patient and accommodate the patient's wishes whenever possible.

Consistency

Another factor known to affect adherence is provider consistency. The adolescent whose clinic care may be provided by any one of several different physicians or other health-care professionals is not as likely to adhere to the regimen as the patient seeing only one physician and/or professional team.

Treatment Regimen

The regimen should be as simple as possible. The more complex it is, the less likely the adolescent will follow it. For example, regimens that require frequent self-monitoring of blood glucose (SMBG) and complicated insulin dose manipulations are much less likely to be adhered to than simple regimens requiring less time commitment from the adolescent. However, the physician should never diminish the importance of frequent SMBG in management.

Testing and Record Keeping

Diabetic adolescents and their parents frequently disagree about testing and record keeping. At each clinic visit, the physician should negotiate with the adolescent on the type and frequency of self-monitoring as well as the kind of records to be maintained. The parents and the adolescent should be informed about the various monitoring techniques and their advantages and disadvantages.

When teaching the adolescent about monitoring, the physician should emphasize that it is done primarily *for the patient's own benefit* not for the parents or physician. The foot-in-the-door approach may be helpful. The physician should ask how much self-monitoring the adolescent believes will permit top-notch diabetes control and then ask how much monitoring he/she is actually willing to do. This information should be shared with the parents and should be well documented both in clinic records and in written instructions to the patient. At the next clinic visit, the patient's success at following the plan is used as a starting point for discussion.

Periodically, the adolescent patient will refuse to do any monitoring; however, even at this point, the physician should not give up. Instead, renegotiate: one urine test per week for ketones is better than not testing at all. (Of course, both patient and parents should be told to call the physician if the test is positive.)

Obviously, one urine test per week is suboptimal diabetes care, but if the adolescent will perform that one task, another can be added at the next clinic visit. This step-by-step approach often yields good results, but progress may be slow.

COMMON PROBLEMS AND ISSUES

Alcohol and Drugs

Some adolescents experiment with alcohol and drugs. This behavior may be an expression of adolescent rebellion and independence, or it may reflect peer pressure. The physician has a responsibility to discuss these issues with patients (Box 31). Without sounding overly authoritarian or judgmental, the physician should explain precisely how drugs and alcohol can affect diabetes. The increased dangers of hypoglycemia with alcohol ingestion should be emphasized. For the adolescent patient whose use of drugs or alcohol appears to be more than simple experimentation, prompt referral for counseling is indicated.

Reproduction

All reproductive-age females with diabetes should be told that it is important to control diabetes *before conception.* Adolescent patients and their parents should have ready access to birth control information.

Prospective spouses of diabetic adolescents should be encouraged to attend clinic visits. In addition, it may be useful to schedule a series of diabetes education sessions for the couple before marriage.

Driving Privileges

Poorly controlled diabetes is associated with fluctuations in blood glucose levels. For safety, the physician should recommend that parents link driving privileges to at least reasonable control of diabetes. For the same reason, the adolescent who drives a motor vehicle should wear a medical identification necklace or bracelet. Furthermore, the physician should remind parents that in controlling the adolescent's access to a motor vehicle, they have a powerful tool for improving adherence to care.

Recurrent Diabetic Ketoacidosis

Diabetic ketoacidosis (DKA) is a life-threatening, usually preventable, complication of diabetes in adolescents. Most cases are associated with poor patient adherence to diabetes care and poor psychosocial adjustment. Recurrent ketoacidosis requires careful evaluation and, if appropriate, prompt referral for counseling.

Participation in Sports

Diabetic adolescents can safely participate in most sports. However, the diabetic athlete should be taught how to adjust food in relation to activity and how to adapt the diabetes regimen to changes in schedule dictated by participation in sports (see **Exercise,** p. 58). Occasionally, it may be necessary for the physician to reassure school officials that the adolescent with diabetes can safely participate in school-sponsored sports.

Misrepresenting Facts

Adolescents with diabetes may misrepresent facts concerning their diabetes care. This is not surprising, given the many care demands and high parental and physician expectations. Most physicians are familiar with instances in which self-monitoring records were falsified. Measurement of glycosylated hemoglobin helps the physician to determine whether home records are accurate.

Box 31. Other Issues in Adolescent Diabetes

Alcohol and drugs
- Use may express rebellion or peer pressure
- Increased danger of hypoglycemia
- Treatment: consider referral for counseling

Sex and marriage
- Well-controlled diabetes before conception
- Ready access to birth control information
- Recommendation: both partners attend clinic and diabetes education sessions

Driving
- Link driving privileges to reasonable control and adherence
- Wear medical identification necklace or bracelet

Recurrent ketoacidosis
- Associated with poor adherence and psychosocial adjustment
- Treatment: prompt referral for counseling

Sports
- Safe participation possible with appropriate adjustment of diabetes regimen
- Physician reassurance of school officials often needed

Misrepresenting facts
- Unrealistic demands and expectations may lead to misrepresentation
- Glycosylated hemoglobin tests may uncover falsified home records
- Recommendation: carefully confront the patient, emphasizing importance of accurate SMBG
- Meal plan tailored to patient with help of dietitian

Parental supervision
- Gradual increase in adolescent responsibilities for care
- Inability to take responsibility may lead to poor control

If physicians find that home records misrepresent the facts, they should confront the adolescent with great care. Forcing a confession serves no useful purpose. Physicians should present this information to the patient in a frank but relaxed and friendly manner. They also should emphasize why accurate home records are important to the patient.

The adolescent may also misrepresent facts concerning eating habits. In this case, enlisting the aid of a dietitian with expertise in diabetes and experience in working with adolescents can be very helpful. The dietitian can work with the adolescent to tailor the meal plan to the patient's food preferences and routines.

The physician should also remind parents that adolescents with diabetes may misrepresent facts to avoid conflicts at home. If adolescents know they will not be punished or criticized for doing poorly with some aspect of care they are more likely to be truthful.

Establishing Independence

Although the major developmental task of adolescence is to establish independence from parents, the process is slow and gradual. The physician should recommend to the parents that they not relinquish diabetes management responsibilities to the adolescent all at once. It is better to gradually increase responsibility. While striving for independence, the adolescent still has some dependency needs and will usually accept some parental supervision. One of the most common causes of poorly controlled diabetes during adolescence is the young patient's inability to assume full responsibility for all aspects of care.

Support Groups and Camps

Support groups for adolescents sponsored by local community and diabetes groups exist in various locales. They may meet regularly, as in the case of "rap" groups, or annually in a camping experience. They are a valuable resource for exchange of information, reinforcement of desirable behavior, and dissipating anxiety that may arise from a sense of being "different."

CONCLUSION

Physicians caring for adolescent patients with diabetes should remember that adolescence is a transient developmental phase and that it may be necessary to make some short-term compromises to achieve long-term successes. The eventual reward is seeing a child who is totally dependent on parents become, in a few years, a capable and independent young adult ready to meet life's challenges, including diabetes care.

BIBLIOGRAPHY

Graber AL, Christman B, Boehm F: Planning for sex, marriage, contraception, and pregnancy. *Diabetes Care* 1:202–203, 1978

Hamburg BA, Inoff GE: Coping with predictable crises of diabetes. *Diabetes Care* 6:409–16, 1983

Hamburg BA, Lipsett LF, Inoff GE, Drash AL (Eds.): *Behavioral and Psychosocial Issues in Diabetes: Proceedings of the National Conference.* Washington, DC, U.S. Govt. Printing Office, 1980, NIH publ. no. 80-1993

Jacobson AM, Leibovich JB: Psychological issues in diabetes mellitus. *Psychosomatics* 25:7–15, 1984

Orr DP, Golden MD, Myers G, Marrero DG: Characteristics of adolescents with poorly controlled diabetes referred to a tertiary care center. *Diabetes Care* 6:179–85, 1983

Simonds JF: Psychiatric status of diabetic youth matched with a control group. *Diabetes* 26:921–25, 1977

Solowiegczyk J, Baker L: Being an adolescent with diabetes. *Diabetes Care* 1:124–25, 1978

Special Problems: The Aged

INTRODUCTION

Medical management of the elderly patient with diabetes differs from that of the younger patient in several important aspects. These include the goals of therapy, the diabetes regimen (insulin, meal plan, and monitoring), and the need to aggressively search for diabetes complications and other disabling conditions.

Several disabilities—generally unique to the elderly, at least in their abundance—may complicate management. Poor dexterity and failing vision may make manipulating a syringe or self-monitoring of blood glucose (SMBG) insuperable tasks. Mild memory impairment or hearing loss may interfere with following physician instructions, and physical and emotional isolation compound any problem.

The diabetes treatment regimen should be kept simple, as outlined below, and should focus on avoiding hypoglycemia and symptomatic hyperglycemia. Maintaining function and general well-being should take precedence over striving for glycemic targets.

ONSET OF DIABETES

Rapid onset of insulin-dependent (type I) diabetes mellitus is unusual in the elderly. The development of insulin deficiency severe enough to mandate insulin therapy may represent a slow evolution of type I diabetes or severe non-insulin-dependent (type II) diabetes. Practically, the differentiation between the two conditions is less important than the decision that insulin is required and sulfonylurea drugs are inappropriate. Attempts to avoid insulin for convenience when it is truly needed may have a disastrous consequence.

DIABETES REGIMEN

For the newly diagnosed patient or the type II patient who is using insulin for the first time, the regimen should entail the minimum number of restrictions and changes in life routine. Previously diagnosed patients accustomed to managing type I diabetes who are still in reasonably good health may continue with their usual regimen unless hypoglycemia develops. Failing health may require simplification of the treatment plan.

Insulin Treatment and Glycemic Goals

Although one injection of insulin each day may not keep the patient symptom free, two injections each day of intermediate-acting insulin often will. Alternatively, a premixed fixed combination of intermediate- and short-acting insulin injected before breakfast and supper may be used.

For many aged patients, normoglycemia is an unrealistic goal. It presents enormous practical difficulties for patients with multiple impairments and increases the likelihood of hypoglycemia. This may aggravate coronary insufficiency and, if it presents as confusion or unconsciousness, it may be misdiagnosed as cerebrovascular accident, vertebrobasilar insufficiency, transient ischemic attack, or syncope. Every elderly diabetic patient has some degree of atherosclerosis, and good medical management of the cardiovascular system should take precedence over normalizing blood glucose.

Monitoring

Because of the high renal threshold in old age, urine glucose tests are not very helpful. A single daily blood glucose level measured before breakfast, which provides a safety check for nocturnal insulin excess or dangerous hyperglycemia, is usually adequate for elderly patients. Multiple daily blood glucose measurements bring little added advantage if a fixed insulin regimen is being followed.

More frequent monitoring, often requiring the help of others, is needed when the patient has symptoms of hypoglycemia or hyperglycemia or is ill. The patient should be given clear instructions on when to call for assistance.

Glycosylated hemoglobin measured several times a year will give the physician an approximation of average glucose control. A glycosylated hemo-

Box 32. A Simple Diabetes Regimen for Aged Patients

Injection and monitoring recommendations

- 2 injections a day of intermediate-acting insulin or a fixed combination of intermediate- and short-acting insulin
- Self-monitoring of blood glucose
  Once a day before breakfast
  More frequently when the patient has *symptoms* of (1) hyperglycemia or (2) hypoglycemia or is *ill*
- HbA_{1c} 10.0%, GHb 12.0% may be acceptable
- Consistent, frequent, simple meals

globin level of less than 10% (HbA_{1c}) or 12% (GHb) may be acceptable in elderly patients (see **Philosophy and Goals,** p. 18).

Nutrition Management

In general, nutritional goals also should be kept modest, avoiding rigid or complex schemes in favor of a balanced consistent meal plan that is as much as possible in concert with long-standing eating habits. The major concern with an elderly patient may not be consuming too much food but too little; therefore, a daily check by a family member or friend is highly advisable to ensure adequate food intake. Deficiencies in protein, vitamins, or minerals may necessitate supplements.

Because of the risk of hypoglycemia, the patient should be strongly advised to avoid fasting for religious reasons.

DIABETES-ASSOCIATED COMPLICATIONS

Both diabetes complications and other sources of disability should be aggressively sought and treated in the elderly patient with diabetes. Maintaining the ability to walk and to see can mean the difference between independent living at home and institutionalization.

Vision Assessment

It is particularly important to identify retinopathy because photocoagulation can save the patient's vision. Other ocular diseases, e.g., senile cataract, macular degeneration, and glaucoma, may be present as well, and they require ophthalmologic consultation. A yearly eye examination should be routine.

In addition to examining the retina, physicians should regularly assess vision with a simple reading acuity chart. Elderly patients may be reluctant to report changes in vision, even if the changes cause them difficulty in seeing marks on syringes or require them to use a magnifying glass to match the colors on their blood glucose or urine glucose test strips. Visually impaired patients may require a family member or visiting nurse to help them with these tasks.

Foot Lesions

More than 50% of nontraumatic amputations occur in diabetic patients, disproportionately often among the elderly. However, these patients may have trouble seeing their feet because of poor vision, have trouble caring for them because of arthritis, and fail to feel injury because of sensory loss.

Prevention of foot ulcers by regular podiatric care and good hygiene is much easier than treatment of established lesions by standard medical care.

No detail is too small when teaching patients to care for their feet. Telling the patient to wipe the foot gently is a simple instruction, but it is this sort of specificity that helps prevent injury and, ultimately, amputation.

Hypertension Assessment

Blood pressure should be assessed frequently and hypertension treated promptly. If possible, beta-adrenergic blocking agents should be avoided because they worsen diabetes control and may cause confusion and disorientation, symptoms easily mistaken for those of hypoglycemia. Nifedipene, a calcium-channel blocker, may have the same effect. All antihypertensive medications should be titrated slowly to avoid hypotension.

Muscle Weakening

Diabetic amyotrophy (bilateral femoral neuropathy) involves a progressive weakening of the muscles of the pelvic girdle and thigh, associated with mild sensory changes. This may be the presenting symptom of diabetes in elderly men. Diabetes should be treated by judicious use of insulin in conjunction with diet. Amyotrophy tends to resolve spontaneously in about 6 to 12 months.

OTHER ASPECTS OF CARE

A Check on Hearing

Physicians should check the hearing of their elderly patients periodically with an informal test (e.g., asking the patient to repeat a few words delivered in a normal voice with the speaker's lips concealed). Elderly patients with mild to moderate hearing loss may be embarrassed to ask a speaker to repeat what has been said or may be unaware of their deficit, believing that others are mumbling, the television volume is too low, etc. Too often, the physician attributes the resulting failure in following treatment instructions to "contrariness" or senile dementia. If hearing loss is detected, the patient should be referred to a specialist.

Mental Status

In appraising mental status, the physician should consider benign or reversible sources of confusion, e.g., hypoglycemia, drugs, or poor hearing. Distinguishing organic from other causes is crucial in evaluating the elderly patient.

Social Status

Compared with younger people, elderly patients are more likely to live alone and to lack ready help from others. Hence, it may be difficult for them to shop, prepare meals, or attend to diabetes care. The physician should become acquainted with the support system of each patient, and family members should be encouraged to provide assistance. Community services such as Meals on Wheels and the Visiting Nursing Association may offer needed nutritional and medical services.

CHECKUP FREQUENCY

Physicians should examine their elderly patients with diabetes frequently, preferably about once every 3 months. At each visit, the physician should check eyes and feet and review details of care. Instructions should be written clearly and concisely. As with younger patients, the physician should periodically ask the aged patient to demonstrate techniques such as insulin injection, foot care, and blood testing.

CONCLUSION

Special effort must be made to meet the needs of older diabetic patients if they are to lead a meaningful life. Goals for glycemic control may be relaxed so that hypoglycemia is avoided, if possible. Vascular complications of aging and/or diabetes should be carefully sought. Individualization is of utmost importance, because age in years is *not* synonymous with aging or loss of vigor.

BIBLIOGRAPHY

Miller Leona V: Managing the elderly patient with diabetes. *Clin Diabetes* 3:73–90, 1985

Tattersall RB: Diabetes in the elderly: a neglected area? *Diabetologia* 27: 167–73, 1984

Complications

Highlights
Complications

RETINOPATHY

Retinopathy in patients with type I diabetes rarely occurs before the 5th year of the disease and reaches a prevalence of 50% by the 10th year. By the 15th year, 50% of patients have proliferative retinopathy.

The clinician should evaluate the retinas of diabetic patients, using the direct ophthalmoscope, at each physical examination or at least annually. Examination through dilated pupils should be performed once a year. Indications for ophthalomological referral can be found on page 113.

Lesions typical of background retinopathy, preproliferative retinopathy, proliferative retinopathy, and macular edema are described on pages 109–112.

High-risk characteristics greatly increase the risk of blindness. If present, photocoagulation is mandatory. High-risk characteristics are listed on page 110.

Retinal photography and intravenous fluorescein angiography should be reserved for certain conditions (p. 112).

Treatment for diabetic retinopathy can be highly effective in preserving or salvaging vision. Treatment modalities include

- panretinal photocoagulation (p. 112),
- focal laser photocoagulation (p. 113), and
- vitrectomy (p. 113).

Medical therapies are discussed on pages 113–114.

NEPHROPATHY

About 30 to 40% of patients affected by type I diabetes will eventually develop end-stage renal failure.

Possible mechanisms by which diabetes damages the kidney are discussed on page 117. Elevated blood glucose, a genetic propensity, or increased renal blood flow have been proposed.

Renal function should be monitored regularly in all patients with type I diabetes (Box 33, p. 117).

Patients with microalbuminuria are at higher risk for developing renal insufficiency and may benefit from more intensive follow-up and therapy. When clinically detectable proteinuria has developed, the long-term prognosis is guarded.

Management of diabetic nephropathy consists of minimizing factors known to accelerate the natural progression of renal disease or factors that may otherwise jeopardize the kidney and of appropriately responding to changing insulin needs (Box 34, p. 118, and Box 35, p. 119).

Aggressive treatment of hypertension is the only therapy that slows the progression of established diabetic nephropathy. Antihypertensive agents are discussed on pages 118–119.

If end-stage renal failure ensues, two options are available—dialysis or renal transplantation (p. 121). The pros and cons of the procedures should be discussed with the patient and his/her family well before end-stage renal failure.

NEUROPATHY

Diabetic neuropathy is classified into a set of discrete clinical syndromes, each with a characteristic presentation and clinical course (Box 36, p. 123). These **syndromes overlap clinically and often occur simultaneously.**

Distal symmetrical polyneuropathy is the most commonly observed form of diabetic neuropathy (p. 124). It may be accompanied by impaired sensation or excruciating pain.

Patients with chronic unrecognized neuropathy may present with late complications, e.g., foot ulceration or foreign objects embedded in the foot. **Feet should be examined at every office visit, and appropriate treatment**

should be initiated if necessary. Infection must always be treated aggressively.

Treatment for diabetic distal symmetrical polyneuropathy is symptomatic, palliative, and supportive, with primary emphasis on preventing the late complications.

Persistent and severely painful neuropathy has been treated with various drugs, including standard analgesics and drugs normally used to treat pain in other conditions, except that narcotics are avoided.

Although autonomic neuropathy produces diffuse subclinical dysfunction, autonomic symptoms are usually confined to one or two organ systems, producing the discrete autonomic syndromes listed in Box 38, page 127. Management guidelines are presented on page 128.

Sexual dysfunction in men with diabetes may be psychogenic, endocrine, vascular, drug or stress related, or neuropathic. Guidelines for management are discussed on page 128.

Other dysfunctions related to autonomic neuropathy include diabetic cystopathy and hypoglycemic unawareness.

Mononeuropathies comprise neural deficits corresponding to the distribution of single or multiple peripheral nerves.

MACROVASCULAR COMPLICATIONS

Coronary heart disease, peripheral vascular disease, and cerebrovascular disease are more common, tend to occur at an earlier age, and tend to be more extensive and severe in people with diabetes.

Many deaths result from the interaction of diabetes and hypertension, hypercholesterolemia, and cigarette smoking.

Physicians should systematically assess patients for risk factors and signs of atherosclerotic cardiovascular disease. **A program for modifying risk factors should be started if appropriate.**

Guidelines for treatment of cerebrovascular disease, coronary heart disease, and peripheral vascular disease appear on page 132.

LIMITED JOINT MOBILITY

Limited joint mobility (LJM) is a potentially important clinical marker for diabetes complications such as retinopathy, nephropathy, neuropathy, and other disorders. Glycosylation of tissue proteins may be responsible for LJM.

LJM may occur in children or adults, is painless, and causes minimal disability. It is marked by a scleroderma-like stiffness of the skin and joints; ultimately, all joints may be affected.

Patients found to have LJM should be carefully examined for complications, e.g., retinopathy, nephropathy, neuropathy, hypertension, and hepatomegaly.

GROWTH

Subtle abnormalities of growth and development affect 5 to 10% of youngsters with type I diabetes mellitus and usually result from inadequate metabolic control.

Signs of growth abnormalities include a lag in height or weight or a falling away from the patient's previously established growth curves (Figure 16, p. 135).

Children most likely to be affected are those with the earliest onset of diabetes and the worst glycemic control. Boys are two or three times more likely to be affected than girls.

To detect growth abnormalities, the physician should plot height and weight on standard growth charts at each office visit. Other growth-impairing conditions should be considered in assessing growth abnormalities (Figure 17, p. 136; Table 21, p. 137).

Retinopathy

INTRODUCTION

Diabetic retinopathy is one of the four most common causes of blindness in the United States and is a major cause of visual disability. Several surveys suggest that a person with diabetes has a 5 to 10% chance of becoming blind.

Retinopathy in patients with insulin-dependent (type I) diabetes mellitus rarely occurs before the 5th year of the disease but reaches a prevalence of 50% by the 10th year. By the 15th year, 50% of patients have proliferative retinopathy, in which new blood vessels develop from the retinal circulation, with a substantial risk of severe hemorrhage and traction detachment of the retina. Puberty appears to be an independent determinant of diabetic retinopathy, which rarely occurs before this time, regardless of diabetes duration.

EYE EXAMINATION

Because diabetic retinopathy appears primarily in the posterior retina within a few optic disk diameters of the optic nerve head (disk) and the macula, most lesions are readily seen by the nonophthalmologist with the monocular direct ophthalmoscope. Every physician should learn how to use this instrument.

Visualization of the retina is enhanced by dilating the pupils, which is easily accomplished in most patients with one drop each of 2.5% phenylephrine hydrochloride and 1% tropicamide. This procedure carries little risk in younger people. Angle-closure glaucoma, a major complication, is a rare disorder in any age group and is virtually nonexistent before age 40 yr. Blurred near vision and sensitivity to bright lights (requiring the use of dark glasses) are temporary inconveniences, lasting only a few hours.

CLINICAL FINDINGS IN DIABETIC RETINOPATHY

Background Retinopathy

The earliest lesion visible through the ophthalmoscope is the *microaneurysm,* a grapelike dilation of capillary-size blood vessels. Ophthalmoscopically, microaneurysms look like tiny red dots. *Dot hemorrhages* may be indistinguishable from microaneurysms unless specialized techniques such as fluorescein angiography are used, but *blot hemorrhages* are easily recognized because they are larger (Figure 5).

Preproliferative Retinopathy

Multiple clustered blot hemorrhages suggest progression to the preproliferative stage because they indicate that substantial portions of the capillary circulation have become nonfunctional, i.e., are nonperfused. It is believed that new blood vessels are formed as a result of the retina's great metabolic need for oxygen and other nutrients supplied by the bloodstream. According to this hypothesis, areas of retinal nonperfusion call forth an angiogenic substance that stimulates the growth of abnormal new blood vessels.

Other preproliferative lesions include *cotton-wool spots,* which are white, usually fluffy-appearing, lesions within the retina that look like puffs of cotton and indicate localized arteriolar closure. In addition, veins may appear *dilated, tortuous, and irregular in caliber. Intraretinal microvascular abnormalities* are another sign of preproliferative retinopathy. These small loops of fine vessels usually extend from a major artery or vein and probably represent early new vessel formation within the retina.

Proliferative Retinopathy

Proliferative diabetic retinopathy involves the formation of new blood vessels, extending from within the retinal substance onto the inner surface of the retina or into the vitreous cavity. These commonly occur on the optic nerve head, where they are called *new vessels on the disk* (NVD) (Figure 6), or elsewhere in the retina, usually extending from major vessels, where they are called *new vessels elsewhere* (NVE). New vessels carry a substantial risk of rupture with hemorrhage or of producing retinal detachment from the tractional forces exerted by the accom-

Figure 5. Early Diabetic Retinopathy

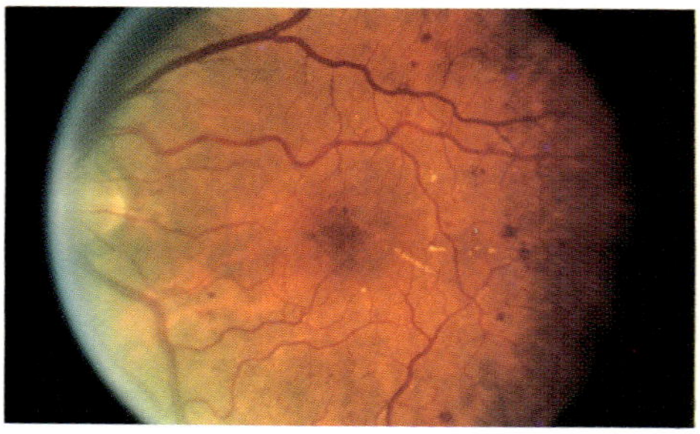

Fundus of patient's left eye is shown, with optic nerve head at *far left* and center of macula appearing as darker zone at *center.* Note scattered microaneurysms and dot hemorrhages and minimal amount of lipid to right of (temporal to) center of macula.

Figure 6. Neovascularization of Disk

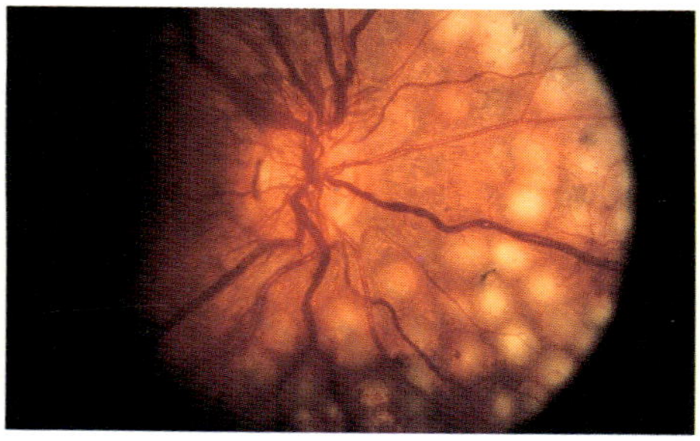

Neovascularization of this extent (greater than ~33% of the disk area) is one of high-risk characteristics for progression to severe blindness during next 3 yr. *White marks* surrounding optic disk at *right* are laser burns, placed in pattern used for panretinal photocoagulation.

Figure 7. Preretinal Hemorrhage

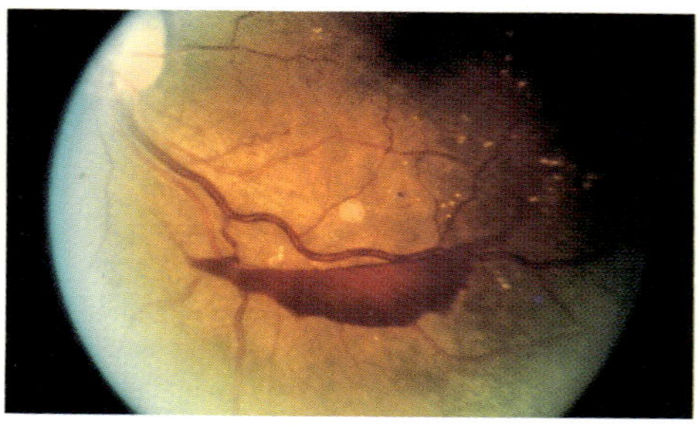

Layered out between posterior face of vitreous gel and inner surface of retina, hemorrhage forms typical boat-shaped configuration. Preretinal hemorrhages may assume other shapes as well. Compact form of hemorrhage, its sharply defined borders, and its location in front of retinal vessels indicate that this is a preretinal, not intraretinal, hemorrhage. Preretinal or vitreous hemorrhages strongly suggest presence of neovascularization.

Figure 8. Diabetic Macular Edema

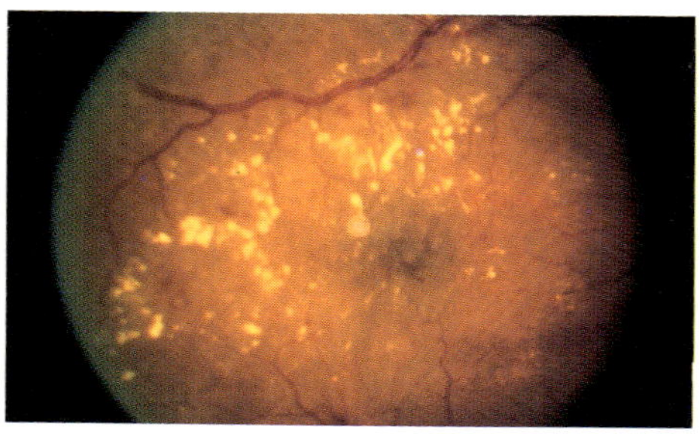

Macular region of right eye is shown. There is much lipid, most of which forms rings (circinate retinopathy). Lipid does not yet involve center of macula. In this monocular view, thickening (edema) of retina cannot be appreciated, especially in centers of lipid rings, but this would be evident by stereoscopic ophthalmoscopy or photographs.

panying strands of fibrous tissue on the thin tissue-paper–like retina.

Certain findings have been termed *high-risk characteristics* (HRCs) by the national Diabetic Retinopathy Study (DRS), a large-scale randomized controlled clinical trial completed in 1981. The presence of HRC increases an eye's risk of blindness (<5/200 vision) to 30 to 50% within 3 to 5 years of detection if appropriate treatment is not given.

High-risk characteristics include

- NVD greater than about 25% of the optic disk area,
- any NVD with preretinal or vitreous hemorrhage, and
- NVE equal to or greater than 50% of the disk area (totaled for the entire retina) with preretinal or vitreous hemorrhage (Figure 7).

When HRCs are present, photocoagulation therapy is mandatory.

Diabetic Macular Edema

Macular edema involves swelling of the central portion of the retina, the macula, which occupies an area of about 5 disk diameters just temporal to the optic nerve head (Figure 8). Visual acuity is decreased in this condition, particularly when the center of the macula (the fovea centralis) is involved. Macular edema cannot be diagnosed by the direct ophthalmoscope because the monocular viewing system of this instrument does not allow the stereoscopic vision necessary to determine retinal swelling. However, the presence of lipid hard exudates—yellowish-white, often glistening deposits of round or irregular shape lying within the retina, usually in the macular region—strongly suggests macular edema. This is particularly true if the exudates assume a ring-shaped, or circinate, configuration.

Sometimes, in far-advanced (usually proliferative) diabetic retinopathy, new vessels may also form on the surface of the iris and extend into the "angle" of the anterior chamber of the eye, where the cornea and iris come together (Figures 9–12). Here, fibrous scar tissue extending from the new vessels may block the outflow of aqueous humor from the eye, causing a tremendous rise in intraocular pressure ("neovascular glaucoma"), severe pain, and loss of vision.

EVALUATION

The clinician should evaluate the retinas of diabetic patients with the direct ophthalmoscope at each physical examination or at least annually.

Patients with type I diabetes should have an annual detailed ocular examination after 5 years of diabetes; the examination need not be done before puberty. The examination should be done by an eye-care specialist certified to perform

- determination of visual acuity in each eye,
- refraction if visual acuity is impaired,
- gross external examination of the eyes,
- evaluation of ocular motility,
- examination of the anterior segments of the eyes by slit-lamp biomicroscopy,
- examination of the retinas with monocular direct and binocular indirect ophthalmoscopy after dilation of the pupils,
- slit-lamp ophthalmoscopy to exclude macular edema, and
- in adult patients, measurement of intraocular pressures, preferably by applanation tonometry.

Some *examinations should be carried out only for specific indications.* These include retinal photography, which is used to document special lesions, and intravenous fluorescein angiography. In this test, a fluorescent dye is injected into the antecubital vein, and rapid-sequence photography of the retinal circulation is carried out with special colored filters in front of the photoflash unit and in front of the film plane of the camera. Both eyes are typically evaluated at a single injection sequence; it is never necessary to perform two separate angiograms to evaluate each eye individually.

Fluorescein angiography is clinically useful to plan photocoagulation treatment for macular edema. Although it is more sensitive than ophthalmoscopy or color photography for detecting very early lesions of retinopathy, the minute lesions thus detected are rarely critical for making decisions regarding treatment. *Therefore, intravenous fluorescein angiography should not be used as a screening test in the annual ocular examination of diabetic patients.* Guidelines for care and referral are described in Box 32.

TREATMENT

Clinicians should always refer patients for treatment to an ophthalmologist, preferably one who is an expert in retinal disease. If laser treatment (described below) has been recommended, the clinician should check that the treatment has been implemented.

Photocoagulation

Panretinal Photocoagulation

The main way to treat diabetic retinopathy today is by argon-laser photocoagulation. For patients with proliferative retinopathy and high-risk characteristics, panretinal photocoagu-

Figure 9. More Severe Preproliferative Diabetic Retinopathy

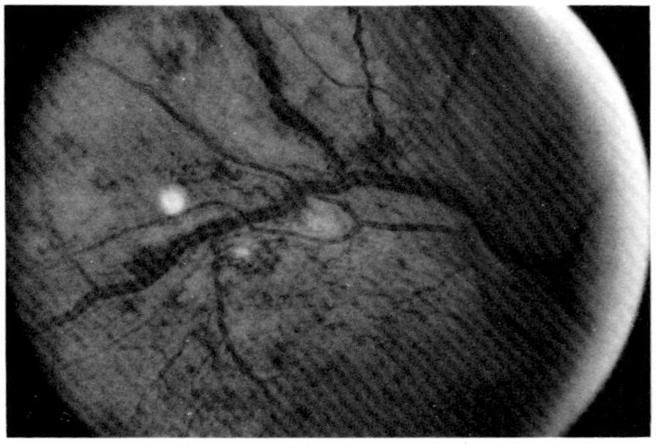

Note markedly dilated and irregular veins. Vein extending from center to 11-o'clock border of photograph looks like string of sausages. There are multiple blot hemorrhages, and 2 cotton-wool spots just below major vein in *center*. Fan-shaped tuft of fine vessels just above major vein (*right center*) may represent early neovascularization. Round, bright white spot above major vein (*left center*) is photographic artifact.

Figure 10. Proliferative Diabetic Retinopathy

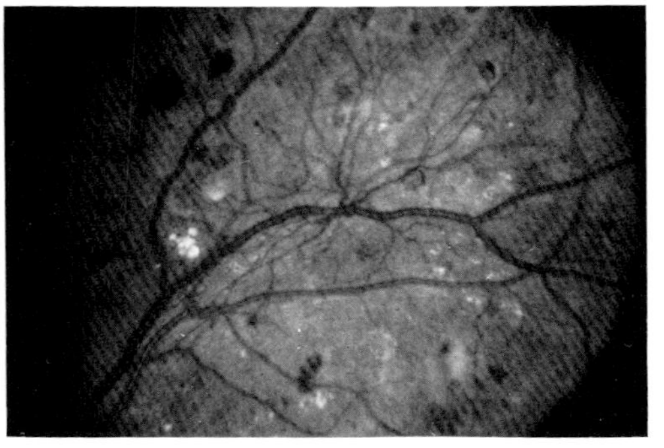

Long fine sprigs of flat neovascularization "elsewhere" (i.e., not on optic disk; also called NVE) arise in fan shape from major vein in *center*. Blot hemorrhages are in *upper left*.

Figure 11. Proliferative Diabetic Retinopathy

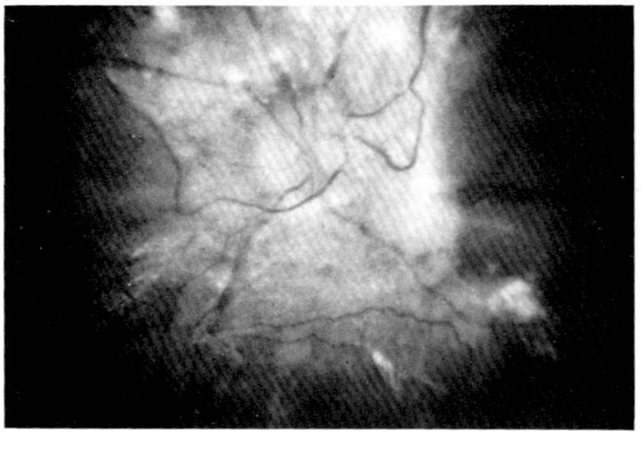

Extensive fibroglial proliferation extends from optic disk, which is dimly seen in *center*. Retinal vessels are bent at right angles by traction from proliferation. Retina is partly detached, with severe loss of vision.

Figure 12. Neovascularization of Iris

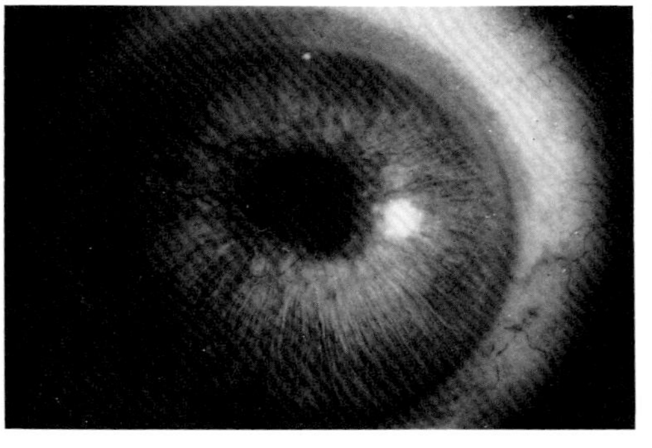

This occurs in far-advanced usually proliferative diabetic retinopathy. Blood vessels are usually not visible on surface of iris, and extensive branching vessels of thick caliber, visible to *left* of pupil, are highly abnormal. They often grow to iris periphery, into anterior chamber angle, which they occlude by accompanying tough fibrous tissue and by hemorrhage and scar formation between root of iris and inner surface of cornea. This produces extreme elevation of intraocular pressure, pain, and blindness. Pupil is irregular partly by contraction because of fibrous tissue and partly because of formation of posterior synechiae, or scars between pupillary border of iris and underlying ocular lens.

lation with the argon laser is standard therapy, based on DRS results.

In this procedure, a series of 1200 to 1600 (or sometimes more) laser burns, 500 micrometers in diameter and spaced one-half burn diameter apart, are placed throughout the midperipheral retina, avoiding the macular region. The DRS demonstrated that this procedure reduced the rate of progression to blindness by 50% in eyes with high-risk characteristics over a 5-year follow-up period.

Many eyes with proliferative retinopathy short of high-risk characteristics or with preproliferative retinopathy are also receiving panretinal photocoagulation, but the efficacy of this treatment in such cases is unproven. The value of panretinal photocoagulation (or of "mild" panretinal photocoagulation, in which 450 to 650 burns are placed around the retina, with much wider spacing than in the standard treatment protocol) in these circumstances is being evaluated in the Early Treatment Diabetic Retinopathy Study (ETDRS), another large-scale randomized, controlled clinical trial. Panretinal photocoagulation also appears to reduce the risk of neovascular glaucoma in eyes with severe retinopathy.

"Focal" Photocoagulation

Diabetic macular edema is currently treated by focal argon-laser photocoagulation. With this technique, leaking microaneurysms and other vascular abnormalities in the macular region, determined by fluorescein angiography, are treated by direct application of small (50- to 100-μm) laser burns. The ETDRS recently showed that this treatment reduced the rate of visual loss from diabetic macular edema by 50% over a 3-year follow-up period.

Box 32. Guidelines for Care

Routine care by physician

- Examine retinas with direct ophthalmoscope at every visit

Referral to eye-care specialist

- Examine retinas through dilated pupils once a year (this need not be done before puberty)

Referral to ophthalmologist

- At the beginning of pregnancy or if planning pregnancy within 12 months
- Immediate referral is *mandatory* (preferably to an ophthalmologist specializing in retinal disease) if any of the following are present.
  - New vessels on the disk (NVD) greater than ~25% of the optic disk area
  - Any NVD with preretinal or vitreous hemorrhage
  - New vessels elsewhere (NVE) ≥50% of the disk area with preretinal or vitreous hemorrhage
- Macular edema (suggested by hard exudates within the macula)
- Reduced vision from any cause
- Immediate referral is *strongly urged* when the following are present.
  - Proliferative retinopathy less than high-risk characteristics
  - Preproliferative retinopathy with:
    dilated irregular veins
    cotton-wool spots
    multiple dot and blot hemorrhages
    intraretinal microvascular abnormalities

Vitrectomy

Vitrectomy is a surgical procedure used to (1) remove vitreous humor filled with blood, (2) cut fibrous traction bands, (3) peel contractile fibrous membranes from the inner retinal surface, and (4) repair some types of complex retinal detachments. It is particularly effective in certain cases of advanced proliferative diabetic retinopathy. Although it can often restore useful vision to eyes that would otherwise be blind, vitrectomy is usually used only in severely diseased eyes, and recovery to near-normal vision after this surgery is the exception, not the rule.

Medical Therapy

Hypertension

It is important to maintain normal blood pressure levels in diabetic patients with retinopathy because of evidence that diabetic retinopathy progresses more rapidly in patients with uncontrolled hypertension than in those whose blood pressure is normal.

Therapies Under Evaluation

Several medical treatments of diabetic retinopathy are being evaluated but as yet are of unproven value.

Aspirin (650 mg/day) is being tested in the ETDRS because it inhibits platelet aggregation. Platelet microthrombi have been proposed as a factor in the cause of diabetic retinopathy.

There is some evidence from animal experiments that a class of drugs called *aldose reductase inhibitors* is useful in preventing or reducing the progression of diabetic retinopathy. By inhibiting aldose reductase, these drugs prevent the enzymatic conversion of glucose to sorbitol, a reaction that is augmented in hyperglycemic states and may result in damage to certain highly susceptible cells, possibly including those of retinal blood vessels. Several clinical trials are evaluating the effectiveness of aldose reductase inhibitors in preventing or slowing the progression of diabetic retinopathy.

The ability of *intensive insulin therapy* to prevent diabetic retinopathy remains controversial (see **Philosophy and Goals,** p. 15). The efficacy of long-term intensive insulin therapy in preventing or slowing the progression of diabetic retinopathy is being evaluated in the Diabetes Control and Complications Trial (DCCT).

Hypophysectomy, performed surgically or by radiation, has been used in a few centers to attempt to halt the progression of severe proliferative diabetic retinopathy that has resisted photocoagulation. Although some studies have suggested a beneficial effect, the value of hypophysectomy in such situations is unproven. In addition, the procedure entails considerable morbidity and mortality.

CONCLUSION

Diabetic retinopathy is a common complication of long-term type I diabetes mellitus that ranks as a leading cause of blindness and visual disability. Although current treatment strategies cannot prevent or cure this complication, there is excellent evidence that they can substantially retard its progression when used appropriately and at the right time. Accordingly, careful evaluation of the ocular fundus of diabetic patients by the primary-care physician, with periodic referral to the ophthalmologist, is a standard of care for all patients with diabetes mellitus.

BIBLIOGRAPHY

Diabetic Retinopathy Study Research Group: Photocoagulation treatment of proliferative diabetic retinopathy: clinical application of Diabetic Retinopathy Study (DRS) findings. *Ophthalmology* 88:583–600, 1981 (DRS rep. no. 8)

Diabetic Retinopathy Vitrectomy Study Research Group: Early vitrectomy for severe vitreous hemorrhage in diabetic retinopathy. *Arch Ophthalmol* 103:1644–52, 1985

Early Treatment Diabetic Retinopathy Study Research Group: Treatment techniques and clinical guidelines for photocoagulation of diabetic macular edema. *Ophthalmology* 94:761–74, 1987 (ETDRS rep. no. 2)

Frank RN: On the pathogenesis of diabetic retinopathy. *Ophthalmology* 91:626–34, 1984

Frank RN: Diabetic retinopathy: current concepts of evaluation and treatment. *Clin Endocrinol Metab* 15: 933–69, 1986

Nephropathy

INTRODUCTION

About 30 to 40% of patients affected by insulin-dependent (type I) diabetes mellitus will eventually develop end-stage renal failure and require dialysis. About one in every four individuals starting dialysis has diabetes, and at least half of these have type I diabetes.

CLINICAL SYNDROME

In its fully established form, diabetic nephropathy is a distinct clinical entity characterized by proteinuria, hypertension, edema, and renal insufficiency, and it occurs in patients with long-standing (usually >10 yr) diabetes mellitus. The most consistent finding is proteinuria, which may be accompanied by hypoalbuminemia and hypercholesterolemia (nephrotic syndrome).

Histopathologic Changes

Three classes of renal histopathologic changes characterize diabetic nephropathy: (1) glomerulosclerosis; (2) structural vascular changes, particularly in the small arterioles; and (3) tubulointerstitial disease. Glomerular damage, e.g., mesangial expansion and basement membrane thickening, is the most characteristic feature of diabetic nephropathy and most often takes the form of diffuse scarring of entire glomeruli. The tubulointerstitial changes interfere with potassium ion and hydrogen ion secretion and may be at least partly responsible for the hyperkalemia and metabolic acidosis that accompany diabetic renal disease.

NATURAL HISTORY OF DIABETIC NEPHROPATHY

When diabetes is first diagnosed, the glomerular filtration rate (GFR) and renal blood flow are characteristically elevated, and there is typically a corresponding increase in kidney weight and size. The serum creatinine and urea nitrogen concentrations are slightly reduced because of this renal hyperfiltration. Although a slight increase in urine protein is common if a patient initially presents in diabetic ketoacidosis, once glycemia is well regulated by insulin therapy, proteinuria disappears and remains absent for many years.

At the onset of clinical diabetes, the renal histology is normal despite renal hypertrophy. However, within 2 to 3 years, many kidneys demonstrate some histological evidence of mesangial expansion and basement membrane thickening. GFR and renal blood flow remain elevated, and proteinuria is not detectable. Figure 13 contains a schematic diagram of diabetic renal disease.

Silent Period

There ensues a long "silent" period (~15 yr) during which there is no laboratory evidence of renal dysfunction. Nonetheless, renal biopsies performed during this period may demonstrate a progressive widespread increase in the characteristic lesions of diabetic nephropathy, despite the fact that GFR usually remains elevated. Microalbuminuria (described below) may be present.

Development of Proteinuria

Although the first laboratory evidence of overt diabetic nephropathy is a dipstick-positive urine test, indicating total albuminuria exceeding 200 to 250 mg in a 24-hour period, abnormalities can sometimes be detected even earlier. Because albumin excretion does not exceed 15 to 25 mg/day in healthy individuals, there is a wide subclinical range (25–250 mg/day) of increased urinary albumin excretion rates that go undetected in routine laboratory testing. The development of more sensitive techniques has permitted the detection of these lower, yet abnormally elevated, albumin excretion rates, referred to as microalbuminuria.

Patients with diabetes and microalbuminuria are at a higher risk for developing renal insufficiency and may benefit from more intensive follow-up and therapy. However, several factors can induce microalbuminuria, including poor diabetes control, stress, infection,

Figure 13. Conceptual Time Frame of Evolution of Nephropathy in Type I Diabetes

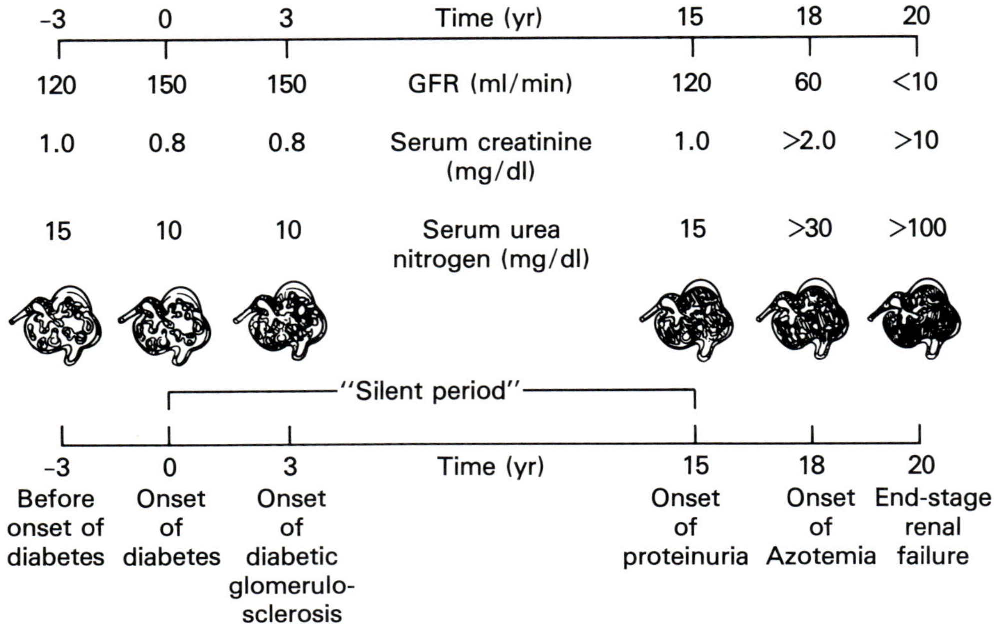

Histologic evidence of diabetic glomerulosclerosis may be present within 3 yr of diagnosis of diabetes. Microalbuminuria may precede frank proteinuria (>250 mg/day) by many years. Onset of routinely detectable proteinuria (dipstick-positive test) is not synonymous with clinical evidence of nephrotic syndrome or azotemia. Silent period is variable, as is entire time frame of proposed schema. GFR, glomerular filtration rate.

hypertension, and exercise. These must be excluded before drawing inferences from the presence of microalbuminuria.

Long-Term Prognosis

When clinically detectable proteinuria has developed (>250 mg/day), the long-term prognosis is guarded. Although the GFR may still be elevated at the onset of proteinuria, it usually declines by about 50% within 3 years, and the serum creatinine and urea nitrogen concentrations become frankly elevated (>2.0 and >30 mg/dl, respectively). Within a mean of 2 years after the serum creatinine becomes elevated (>2.0 mg/dl), 50% of the individuals will have progressed to end-stage renal failure. During this period, uremic symptoms, including drowsiness, lethargy, and nausea, appear and become progressively more pronounced.

Traditionally, it has been considered unusual to observe diabetic nephropathy in the absence of retinopathy, neuropathy, and hypertension. However, the correlation now appears to be especially close only in advanced renal disease. At onset of proteinuria, an estimated 30 to 40% of patients have no retinopathy, 50% have no neuropathy, and 75% have normal blood pressure. As kidney failure progresses, incidence and severity of all three disorders rises markedly, generally in parallel with renal status.

PATHOGENESIS OF DIABETIC NEPHROPATHY

Considerable evidence suggests that diabetic nephropathy is primarily related to the metabolic changes induced by the diabetic state. First, renal changes are initially absent in people biopsied around the time of onset of diabetes.

Second, typical changes of diabetic nephropathy occur in all types of diabetes. Third, diabetic nephropathy appears in various animal models regardless of whether the diabetes is induced or spontaneous, and the damage occurs in both original and transplanted kidneys. Fourth, in these diabetic animals, intensive insulin therapy or islet cell transplantation completely prevents renal histopathologic changes and may reverse early histopathologic abnormalities.

Possible Mechanisms of Damage

The mechanisms by which diabetes damages the kidney remain unknown. It has not been established whether elevated glucose per se or some metabolic event that occurs as a consequence of hyperglycemia is the trigger, and the value of tight diabetes control to prevent the initiation of renal damage is the subject of current study (see **Philosophy and Goals,** p. 16).

A genetic propensity to diabetic nephropathy may also contribute to its development. Thus, it is possible that metabolic disturbances initiate the processes responsible for diabetic nephropathy but that these processes operate on a genetic background that predisposes to diabetic glomerulosclerosis.

One explanation for renal damage may involve the typical increases in GFR and renal blood flow that occur early in the course of diabetes. In animals, these alterations in renal hemodynamics are associated with increased intraglomerular pressures. Although it has not been possible to measure intraglomerular pressure in human beings, it has been suggested that glomerular hypertension, regardless of what derangements or predispositions lead up to it, is the ultimate mediator of kidney damage in diabetic nephropathy. If so, measures aimed at reversing the resulting hemodynamic changes may prove useful in slowing the progression of renal disease in human diabetes.

MANAGEMENT OF DIABETIC NEPHROPATHY

Beginning at diagnosis of diabetes, renal status of all patients with diabetes should be monitored as outlined in Box 33. Hypertension should be aggressively treated.

Box 33. Monitoring Renal Function

In the first 5 yr of diabetes, a routine urinalysis with a check for proteinuria should be obtained at each visit. Serum creatinine and urea nitrogen concentrations should be measured at least once a year if proteinuria is present.

Beyond 5 yr or in the postpubertal patient, in addition to the above tests, 24-h urine should be collected at least once a year to quantitate total protein excretion. If possible, tests for microalbuminuria should be conducted.

Once overt proteinuria or elevated serum creatinine/urea nitrogen is detected, renal function should be monitored at least 2–3 times a year. Consultation with a nephrologist is necessary to plot a long-term therapeutic strategy and to discuss the possibility and implications of renal failure with the patient.

Currently, the management of diabetic nephropathy is largely preventive and supportive. It consists of minimizing factors that are known to accelerate the natural progression of renal disease or that may otherwise jeopardize the kidney, and it consists of appropriately responding to changing insulin needs (Boxes 34 and 35). If end-stage renal failure ensues, two options are available: dialysis or renal transplantation.

HYPERTENSION

Hypertension is the single most important factor shown to accelerate the progression of established diabetic nephropathy and contributes to other causes of diabetes-related morbidity and mortality such as retinopathy and heart disease. *Aggressive treatment of hypertension is the only therapeutic intervention shown to slow the progression of established renal disease.* Therefore, it is paramount that the patient with diabetes have blood pressure normalized (120–130/80 mmHg) to the extent possible without compromising cardiac, cerebral, or other organ-system functions. A list of drugs of potential use in treating hypertension in patients with di-

Box 34. Treatment of Diabetic Nephropathy

The following are factors influencing diabetic nephropathy.

- *Hypertension*—the most important factor shown to accelerate progression of renal failure
  - Treatment, diuretic (very volume sensitive) plus antihypertensive agent.
  - Specific antihypertensive drugs are listed in Table 19.
  - Converting-enzyme inhibitors may have a specific effect to preserve renal function.

- *Urinary tract infection:* increased incidence, frequent cultures.

- *Neurogenic bladder:* parasympathetic/alpha-adrenergic–blocking drugs, voiding maneuvers, bladder-neck resection.

- *Intravenous pyelography and other radiographic dyes:* increased evidence of acute renal failure, particularly if heavy proteinuria and renal impairment are present.

- *Blood glucose control*
  - Uremia is associated with insulin resistance and increased insulin requirements.
  - With advanced uremia (glomerular filtration rate 15–20 ml/min), insulin requirements may be decreased because the kidney removes 25% of daily injected insulin and hepatic degradation of insulin is inhibited by uremia.

- *Protein restriction*
  - There are good data on animals and preliminary data on humans indicating that a low-protein diet slows progression of renal disease in nondiabetic individuals with advanced renal insufficiency. A similar beneficial effect has been reported in diabetic patients.
  - It is unknown whether protein restriction, instituted early in renal disease, will prevent or ameliorate progression of either diabetic or nondiabetic nephropathy.

Intensive insulin therapy is of unproven benefit. There is no evidence that tight metabolic control prevents or ameliorates the progression of established renal disease. Whether insulin-pump therapy instituted within the first 1–2 yr after the diagnosis of diabetes mellitus will prevent the development of renal disease remains to be established by prospective trials.

abetes, along with their side effects, is given in Table 19.

Hypertension Therapy

Because hypertension in the diabetic patient is largely volume sensitive, therapy may be initiated with a low-sodium diet and a diuretic. Because many hypertensive individuals with diabetes have some degree of renal insufficiency, a loop diuretic is usually necessary. Thiazide diuretics do not promote diuresis once the serum creatinine has risen to levels greater than 2.0 mg/dl. Also, use of diuretics that inhibit potassium secretion (e.g., spironolactone, triamterene) is not recommended for patients with diabetes because of concern for inducing hyperkalemia.

Angiotensin-Converting–Enzyme Inhibitors

Recent studies suggest that angiotensin-converting–enzyme inhibitors (e.g., enalopril, captopril) are effective in lowering blood pressure in patients with diabetic nephropathy and may also decrease proteinuria. Some evidence shows that they may actually ameliorate the progression of renal disease by specifically decreasing intraglomerular pressure. However, further controlled studies are needed to confirm this.

The major side effect of captopril and enalopril is hyperkalemia, which is of particular concern because patients with type I diabetes may have the syndrome of hyporeninemic hypoaldosteronism. In the presence of low renin, circulating aldosterone levels are decreased, and the renal tubular secretion of potassium

Box 35. Other Threats to Diabetic Kidneys

Several conditions can endanger the kidneys of diabetic individuals, regardless of whether renal insufficiency has come into play. Among them are the following.

Urinary tract infection. Older individuals with diabetes generally have an increased incidence of urinary tract infection. Therefore, for these patients, it is important that a urinalysis be performed on each clinic visit. If white blood cells or bacteriuria are detected, a urine culture should be obtained. Positive cultures should be treated with an appropriate bactericidal antibiotic.

Neurogenic bladder. The development of a neurogenic bladder is common in patients with diabetes, especially if other evidence of autonomic neuropathy is present, and may predispose to infection. Symptoms (frequent voiding, nocturia, incontinence, recurrent urinary tract infections) may be minimal or may mimic those of prostatic hypertrophy. Once suspected, the diagnosis is easily established if a cystometrogram demonstrates a large atonic bladder with low pressure recordings.

If the presence of a neurogenic bladder is confirmed, the patient should receive instruction in the Credé manual voiding maneuver, which should be performed every 6–8 h. Often this will be sufficient to prevent postvoid residual and will decompress the upper urinary tract. If not, parasympathetic agents such as urecholine may be tried. In some people with diabetes, alpha-adrenergic–blocking drugs such as phenoxybenzamine have proven useful. If pharmacologic therapy proves unsuccessful, intermittent straight catheterization should be performed 2–3 times daily.

Intravenous pyelography and other dye studies. Patients with diabetes are at increased risk for acute renal failure after any radiocontrast [intravenous and retrograde pyelography, arteriography, cholangiography, computed tomography (CT) scanning] procedure. Patients with an elevated serum creatinine or proteinuria are at greatest risk. With the judicious use of echography, radionuclide studies, and noncontrast CT scanning, radiocontrast studies are rarely necessary.

If contrast media must be used, a minimum amount of dye should be given, and adequate hydration should be ensured before the dye study. An osmotic diuresis with mannitol should be started before and continued for 24 h after infusion of the radiocontrast medium. Serum creatinine concentration should be checked daily for 2–3 days after the contrast study.

is impaired. Any drug that further impairs aldosterone secretion or action may lead to clinically significant hyperkalemia.

Some patients may experience a precipitous decline in renal function when therapy with angiotensin-converting–enzyme inhibitors begins. Because this appears to be more common in patients with impaired renal function, the physician should determine serum creatinine and potassium levels approximately 1 week after therapy begins. An excessive increase in either level warrants discontinuation of the drug.

Beta-Adrenergic–Blocking Agents

Beta-adrenergic–blocking agents have also proven successful in treating the hypertensive patient with diabetes. However, this class of drugs inhibits hepatic glucose production, which may lead to hypoglycemia, and they may mask many of the warning symptoms of hypoglycemia (sweating is not affected).

Beta-blocking agents also predispose the development of hyperkalemia by inhibiting renin synthesis and impairing potassium uptake by extrarenal tissues. Specific $beta_1$-antagonists should be employed in patients with diabetes because they are less likely to cause hypoglycemia and hyperkalemia.

Calcium-Channel Blockers

This class of drugs is not officially approved for the treatment of hypertension but is being evaluated for this purpose. The drugs are relatively free of side effects and do not cause significant alterations in glucose or lipid metabolism. Because of the high incidence of side effects, reserpine and guanethidine should be used with extreme caution in individuals with diabetes.

Table 19. Potential Complications of Antihypertensive Drugs in Diabetic Patients

DRUG	POTENTIAL COMPLICATIONS
Diuretics	
Potassium losing	Hypokalemia
Thiazides	Hyperglycemia
Loop diuretics	Hyperlipidemia
	Impotence
Potassium sparing	Hyperkalemia
Spironolactone	Impotence
Triamterene	Gynecomastia
Vasodilators	
Hydralazine	Exacerbation of coronary heart disease
Minoxidil	
Sympathetic inhibitors	
Methyldopa	Orthostatic hypotension
Clonidine	Impotence
Guanabenz	Depression
Alpha-adrenergic blockers	
Prazosin	Orthostatic hypotension
Beta-adrenergic blockers	
Nonselective	Cardiac failure
Propranolol	Impaired insulin release with hyperglycemia
Nadolol	
Timolol	Delayed recovery from hypoglycemia
Pindolol	
Cardioselective*	Blunted symptoms of hypoglycemia
Metoprolol	
Atenolol	Hypertension associated with hypoglycemia
	Hyperlipidemia
Angiotensin-converting–enzyme inhibitors	
Captopril	Proteinuria
Enalapril	Hyperkalemia
	Leukopenia/agranulocytosis

*Cardioselectivity may be lost with high doses.

Adapted from Christlieb AR: Treating hypertension in the patient with diabetes. *Med Clin N Am* 66: 1373–88, 1982

OTHER ASPECTS OF TREATMENT

Blood Glucose Control

There is no firm evidence that tight glycemic control through intensive insulin therapy (i.e., insulin pump or multiple injections) can reverse or even slow the progression of established renal disease. One recent well-controlled study in diabetic patients with microalbuminuria has shown that intensified insulin therapy can prevent the development of persistent proteinuria. Whether intensified insulin treatment can prevent or decrease the incidence of new cases of diabetic nephropathy is the subject of current study. Striving for normoglycemia should not be discouraged for motivated individuals with diabetic nephropathy who have no contraindications (e.g., hypoglycemic unawareness) to intensive insulin therapy.

The development of renal insufficiency is associated with insulin resistance, and it is common to observe an increase in insulin requirements. As renal failure worsens (serum creatinine concentration >4–5 mg/dl), the degradation of insulin becomes progressively impaired, and it is not uncommon to see a decrease in the daily insulin dose and/or an increase in hypoglycemic episodes. For these reasons, and because urine glucose tests are unreliable in renal failure, *blood glucose monitoring is required to properly adjust insulin dosage in patients with renal failure.*

Low-Protein Diet

Over the last several years, there has been renewed interest in the use of low-protein diets to prevent the progression of chronic renal failure. Studies in nondiabetic patients with advanced renal failure (creatinine clearance <25 ml/min) have shown that a restricted protein intake (<40–50 g of high-quality protein/day) will have a palliative effect on the progression of renal failure. However, it is not known whether similar beneficial effects will also be observed in nondiabetic patients with less severe degrees of renal insufficiency, and little is known about the value of low-protein diets in patients with diabetic renal disease.

A low-protein diet must be high in carbohydrate and/or fat, and the long-term effects of such a diet on atherosclerotic complications and glycemic control are unknown. Similarly, it is not known whether a low-protein diet can maintain a normal nitrogen balance in a diabetic patient with advanced renal insufficiency. Therefore, the use of low-protein diets in the treatment of diabetic nephropathy should be considered experimental, pending further information concerning their efficacy and safety.

DIALYSIS AND RENAL TRANSPLANTATION

Once end-stage renal failure ensues, prolonging life requires dialysis or a functioning renal transplant. The pros and cons of these procedures should be discussed with patients and their families well in advance of end-stage renal failure. The prospect of needing such measures should never come as a surprise. The ultimate choice among alternatives requires input from the patient, the patient's family, a nephrologist, and the primary-care physician.

A plot of the reciprocal of the serum creatinine (1/serum creatinine) or the creatinine clearance as a function of time is relatively linear and provides a reasonable estimate of how fast renal function is deteriorating. This plot can aid the physician in deciding when to refer the patient to a nephrologist.

Absolute indications for dialysis or transplantation include serum creatinine greater than 8 mg/dl or creatinine clearance of 10 ml/min or less as well as urgent uremic symptoms, e.g., seizures, uremic pericarditis, unresponsive hypertension, and muscle deterioration. More subjective criteria include worsening lethargy, nausea or vomiting, and progressive retinopathy and neuropathy.

Renal Dialysis

Of the various forms of renal dialysis, hemodialysis is the most frequently used in diabetic patients, although various forms of peritoneal dialysis have also been used with success. Some patients using intermittent or continuous ambulatory peritoneal dialysis (CAPD) have insulin included with the dialysate. This procedure often improves blood glucose control because peritoneal insulin delivery is more physiologic than subcutaneous delivery. CAPD also affords a motivated patient the greatest mobility, although its long-term efficacy in comparison to other dialysis techniques is still under study.

Kidney Transplantation

As the success rate of kidney transplantation continues to improve, this procedure is being used more frequently in patients with diabetes. Kidneys donated by first-degree relatives continue to be preferable, although increasing experience with immunosuppressive agents has helped lower the incidence of rejection with tissue-matched cadaver-donated kidneys.

The decision of whether to opt for a transplant is still not one to be taken lightly, and a patient must be well briefed on the chances of failure, as well as the probability (for younger patients) that the new kidney will undergo the same changes that caused the original kidney to fail. Nonetheless, the options available in the event of end-stage renal failure offer greater possibilities than were available even 5 years ago for salvaging quality of life and increasing longevity.

An excellent review of the therapeutic options available to the diabetic patient with end-stage renal failure has been published (see Bibliography, Kjellstrand).

CONCLUSION

End-stage renal disease is a major cause of morbidity and mortality in patients with type I diabetes of longer than 15 years duration. Vigilant monitoring of evolving proteinuria (including microalbuminuria), striving for glycemic control within patient-acceptable goals, aggressive therapy of hypertension, and anticipating the need for dialysis or transplantation, form the cornerstones of management. The primary-care provider is pivotal in integrating available resources, including referral to a nephrologist.

BIBLIOGRAPHY

Kaplan NM, Rosenstock J, Raskin P: A differing view of treatment of hypertension in patients with diabetes mellitus. *Arch Intern Med* 147: 1160–62, 1987

Kjellstrand CM: A comparison of dialysis and transplantation in patients with end stage renal failure of diabetes. In *Diabetic Renal-Retinal Syndrome*. Vol. 3. Friedman EA, L'Esperance FA, Eds. Orlando, FL, Grune & Stratton, 1986, p. 333–40

Mogensen CE, Christensen CK: Predicting diabetic nephropathy in insulin-dependent patients. *N Engl J Med* 311:89–93, 1984

Viberti GC, Walker JD: Diabetic nephropathy: etiology and prevention. *Diabetes Metab Rev*. In press

Viberti GC, Wiseman MJ: The kidney in diabetes: significance of the early abnormalities. *Clin Endocrinol Metab* 15:753–82, 1986

The Working Group on Hypertension in Diabetes: Statement on hypertension in diabetes mellitus. *Arch Intern Med* 147:830–42, 1987

Zatz R, Brenner BM: Pathogenesis of diabetic microangiopathy: the hemodynamic view. *Am J Med* 80:443–53, 1986

Neuropathy

INTRODUCTION

Peripheral neuropathy is one of the most common and troubling chronic complications of diabetes. Virtually all regions of the body can be affected by diabetic neuropathy, which can produce significant impairments alone and in concert with other conditions. Most notably, neuropathic loss of sensation in the foot regularly conspires with infection and/or vascular insufficiency (more common in people with diabetes) to make diabetes the most frequent source of nontraumatic lower-limb amputations in the United States.

OVERVIEW OF NEUROPATHIES

The frequency of diabetic neuropathy parallels duration and severity of hyperglycemia, in both insulin-dependent and non-insulin-dependent (types I and II, respectively) diabetes mellitus. In patients with type I diabetes, it rarely occurs within the first 5 years after diagnosis. Neuropathy also occurs in diabetes caused by pancreatectomy, nonalcoholic pancreatitis, and hemochromatosis and independently in conditions more commonly associated with type I diabetes, e.g., hypothyroidism and pernicious anemia.

Histological Findings

Histologically, there is loss of both large and small myelinated nerve fibers, accompanied by varying degrees of paranodal and segmental demyelination, connective tissue proliferation, and thickening and reduplication of capillary basement membranes with capillary closure. Researchers are investigating several potential pathways by which hyperglycemia (perhaps aided by other metabolic derangements of diabetes) may cause such changes.

Treatment of Neuropathies

There is no known direct treatment for neuropathy. Some investigators see a role for intensified glycemic control in managing or preventing neuropathy, although conclusive substantiating evidence is still pending from controlled clinical trials. Dietary supplements of *myo*-inositol have been suggested based on animal studies, but fragmentary clinical experience has been inconclusive. Aldose reductase inhibitors, which block the accumulation of sorbitol and loss of *myo*-inositol from diabetic nerve and improve nerve conduction in diabetic animals and patients, are undergoing clinical trials in symptomatic neuropathy.

Clinical Syndrome

Diabetic neuropathy is classified into a set of discrete clinical syndromes, each with a characteristic presentation and clinical course (Box 36). Because the syndromes overlap clinically and frequently occur simultaneously, rigid classification of individual cases is often difficult. Identical neurological syndromes occur in other diseases, and other conditions, e.g., occlusive peripheral vascular disease and hysterical conversion reaction, can mimic peripheral neuropathy, resulting in diabetic neuropathy as a diagnosis of exclusion (Box 37).

Box 36. Syndromes of Diabetic Neuropathy

Diffuse neuropathies (common, insidious onset, usually progressive)
- Distal symmetrical sensorimotor polyneuropathy
- Autonomic neuropathy

Focal neuropathies (rare, sudden onset, usually transient)
- Cranial neuropathy
- Radiculopathy
- Plexopathy
- Mononeuropathy/mononeuropathy multiplex
    - Entrapment neuropathy
    - Other mononeuropathies

Box 37. Common Conditions Resembling Various Forms of Diabetic Neuropathy

Distal symmetrical neuropathy
- Inflammatory neuropathies (vasculitic, i.e., systemic lupus erythematosis, polyarteritis, and other connective tissue diseases; sarcoidosis; leprosy)
- Metabolic neuropathies (hypothyroidism, uremic; nutritional; acute intermittent porphyric)
- Toxic neuropathies (alcohol; drugs; heavy metals, e.g., lead, mercury, and arsenic; industrial hydrocarbons)
- Other neuropathies (paraneoplastic; dysproteinemic, amyloid, hereditary)

Autonomic neuropathy
- Idiopathic orthostatic hypotension
- Shy-Drager syndrome (progressive autonomic failure)

Cranial neuropathy
- Carotid aneurysm
- Intracranial mass
- Elevated intracranial pressure

Radiculopathy
- Spinal cord/root compression
- Transverse myelitis
- Coagulopathies
- Shingles

Plexopathy
- Mass lesions
- Coagulopathies
- Cauda equina lesions (femoral neuropathy)

Mononeuropathy/mononeuropathy multiplex
- Compression neuropathies
- Inflammatory (vasculitic) neuropathies
- Hypothyroidism, acromegaly

DISTAL SYMMETRICAL SENSORIMOTOR POLYNEUROPATHY

Distal symmetrical polyneuropathy is the most common form of diabetic neuropathy. Sensory signs and symptoms generally predominate over motor involvement and vary depending on the classes of nerve fibers. Loss of large fibers produces diminished proprioception and light touch, resulting in ataxic gait, unsteadiness, and weakness of intrinsic muscles in the hands and feet. Involvement of small fibers causes diminished pain and temperature sensation, resulting in unrecognized trauma (especially to the feet), accidental burning of the hands, etc.

Typical neuropathic paresthesia (spontaneous uncomfortable sensations) or dysesthesia (contact paresthesia) may accompany both large- and small-fiber involvement. Sensory deficits first appear in the most distal portions of the extremities and spread proximally with disease progression in a "stocking-glove" distribution. In the most advanced cases, vertical bands of sensory deficit develop on the chest when the tips of the shorter truncal nerves become involved (Figure 14).

Occasionally, patients complain of exquisite hypersensitivity to light touch, superficial burning or stabbing pain, or bone-deep aching or tearing pain, usually most troublesome at night. Sometimes, neuropathic pain may become the overriding and disabling feature, especially in small-fiber neuropathy. Both neuropathic pain and paresthesia are thought to reflect spontaneous depolarization of newly regenerating nerve fibers.

Asymptomatic Neuropathy

Many patients with distal symmetrical polyneuropathy remain free of troubling subjective symptoms. In these cases, it may take careful questioning to learn of a patient's subtle feelings of numbness or cold or "dead" feet. Diminished or absent deep tendon reflexes, especially the Achilles tendon reflex, is often an early indication of otherwise asymptomatic neuropathy. However, in the absence of pain or paresthesia, diabetic neuropathy may go unrecognized unless the physician routinely tests foot sensation during office visits.

LATE COMPLICATIONS OF POLYNEUROPATHY

Patients with chronic unrecognized neuropathy may present with late complications, e.g., foot ulceration, foreign objects embedded in the foot, unrecognized trauma to the extremities, or neuroarthropathy (Charcot's joints). All of these conditions are avoidable with proper early diagnosis of neuropathy.

Foot Ulcerations and Infections

Acute foot ulcerations and resulting infections can occur when an individual cannot feel pain due to poorly fitting shoes (a source of penetrating abrasions), a retained foreign body, or accidental trauma (often unintentionally self-inflicted during nail trimming). Plantar ulcers, which form at the callused sites of maximal walking pressure, can result from a combination of motor, cutaneous sensory, and proprioceptive deficits.

Patients with long-standing diabetes and neuropathy are also predisposed to chronic venous stasis ulcers, vascular ulcers due to macrovascular and microvascular insufficiency, and ischemic gangrene.

In a typical sequence of events, imbalance of extensor and flexor muscles in the feet, resulting from impaired proprioception and atrophy of intrinsic extensor muscles, leads to tendon shortening and chronic toe flexion (claw-toe deformity). This in turn shifts weight bearing from the padded ball of the foot to the unprotected metatarsal heads. With pain insensitivity, trauma to the overlying skin goes undetected, producing thick calluses that further concentrate weight bearing over the bony prominences. Splitting and fissuring of the thick callus initiates ulcer formation, further aggravated by infection and vascular insufficiency.

Neuroarthropathy

Neuroarthropathy refers to the joint erosions, unrecognized fractures, demineralization, and devitalization of bones in the foot resulting from the routine daily weight-bearing activities in which neuropathy impairs normal protective proprioceptive and nociceptive functions. The foot may be swollen and red but not necessarily painful, and the problem may be misdiagnosed as cellulitis despite normal white cell count and differential and the absence of fever. The patient may report relatively painless trauma, and initial radiographic examination may be unrevealing, whereas follow-up X rays several days or weeks later may reveal clear traumatic changes. In more advanced cases, devitalization of bone may mimic osteomyelitis, and in the most advanced stages, the foot may look like a "bag of bones."

Figure 14. Distribution of Sensory Loss in Patient With Severe Chronic Diabetic Sensory Polyneuropathy

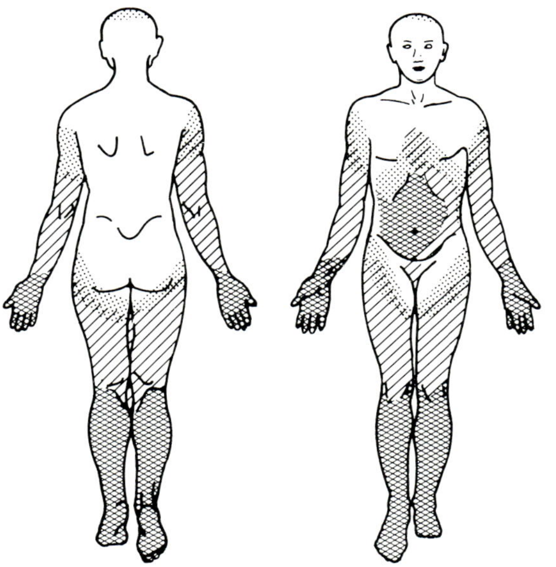

Loss is maximal distally in limbs but also affects anterior trunk and vertex of head. *Hatched lines,* pinprick impaired; *cross-hatched lines,* pinprick absent; *stippled lines,* hyperesthesia. *From* Sabin TD, Geschwind M, Waxman SG: Patterns of clinical deficits in peripheral nerve disease. In *Physiology and Pathophysiology of Axons.* New York, Raven, 1987, p. 431–38

MANAGEMENT OF DISTAL SYMMETRICAL POLYNEUROPATHY AND COMPLICATIONS

Treatment for diabetic distal symmetrical polyneuropathy is symptomatic, palliative, and supportive, with primary emphasis on preventing the late complications.

In most cases, the primary neuropathic symptoms consist of mild intermittent pain or paresthesia. Even severely painful symptoms generally remit spontaneously within a few months in most but not all patients.

Management of Pain

Persistent and severely painful neuropathy has been treated with various drugs, including standard analgesics and

Table 20. Warning Symptoms and Signs of Diabetic Foot Problems

	SYMPTOMS	SIGNS
Vascular	Cold feet Intermittent claudication involving calf or foot Pain at rest, especially nocturnal, relieved by dependency	Absent pedal, popliteal, or femoral pulses Femoral bruits Dependent rubor, plantar pallor on elevation Prolonged capillary filling time (>3–4 s) Decreased skin temperature
Neurologic	Sensory: burning, tingling, or crawling sensations; pain and hypersensitivity; complaints of cold or "dead" feet, unsteady gait Motor: weakness (drop foot) Autonomic: diminished sweating	Sensory: deficits (vibratory and proprioceptive, then pain and temperature perception), hyperesthesia Motor: diminished to absent deep tendon reflexes (Achilles then patellar), weakness Autonomic: diminished to absent sweating
Musculoskeletal	Gradual change in foot shape Sudden painless change in foot shape, with swelling, without history of trauma	Cavus feet with claw toes Drop foot "Rocker-bottom" foot (Charcot's joint) Neuropathic arthropathy
Dermatologic	Exquisitely painful or painless wounds Slow-healing or nonhealing wounds, necrosis Skin color changes (cyanosis, redness) Chronic scaling, itching, or dry feet Recurrent infections (e.g., paronychia, athlete's foot)	Skin Abnormal dryness Chronic tinea infections Keratotic lesions with or without hemorrhage (plantar or digital) Trophic ulcer Hair Diminished to absent Nails Trophic changes Onychomycosis Subungual ulceration or abscess Ingrown nails with paronychia

From Scardina RJ: Diabetic foot problems: assessment and prevention. *Clin Diabetes* 1:1–7, 1983

drugs normally used to treat pain in other conditions, but narcotics are avoided. Subantidepressive doses of amitriptyline or other tricyclic antidepressants, often combined with fluphenazine, are helpful in some but not all patients and should be given a short therapeutic trial. Although not substantiated by controlled clinical trials, anticonvulsive doses of phenytoin or carbamazepine have been used based on their membrane-stabilizing properties. Transcutaneous electrical nerve stimulation has also been used for refractory painful neuropathy.

Because early diagnosis of asymptomatic neuropathy is essential for preventing the late complications, *no physician visit should go by without a thorough examination of the feet.* A listing of neurologic and related symptoms to watch for is given in Table 20.

Callus Formation and Plantar Ulcers

Callus formation over weight-bearing areas indicates the need to consult a podiatrist and/or orthopedist for prescription of corrective footwear to redistribute weight bearing. Plantar ulcers should be managed by eliminating weight bearing either by special walking casts or by bed rest. Refractory and/or recurrent ulcers may be managed by surgical removal of the involved metatarsal. Neuroarthropathy is managed by reduced ambulation and weight bearing as well as cushioned footwear.

Treatment of Infection

Infection must be treated aggressively with appropriate consultation from infectious-disease specialists. Antibiotics effective against anaerobic organisms should be included in the treatment regimen. Vascular bypass surgery or percutaneous angioplasty should be considered if arterial insufficiency is a major contributing factor.

AUTONOMIC NEUROPATHY

Neuropathy can affect virtually any autonomic function in patients with diabetes. Although autonomic neuropathy produces diffuse subclinical dysfunction, autonomic symptoms are usually confined to one or two organ systems, producing the discrete autonomic syndromes listed in Box 38.

Box 38. Syndromes of Autonomic Neuropathy

Cardiovascular autonomic neuropathy
- Resting sinus tachycardia without sinus arrythmia (fixed heart rate)
- Exercise intolerance
- Painless myocardial infarction
- Orthostatic hypotension
- Sudden death

Gastrointestinal autonomic neuropathy
- Esophageal dysfunction
- Autonomic gastropathy and delayed gastric emptying
- Diabetic diarrhea
- Constipation
- Fecal incontinence

Genitourinary autonomic neuropathy
- Erectile impotence
- Retrograde ejaculation with infertility
- Bladder dysfunction

Hypoglycemic unawareness

Sudomotor neuropathy
- Facial sweating
- Heat intolerance
- "Gustatory" sweating

Cardiovascular Autonomic Neuropathy

The earliest clinical signs of cardiovascular autonomic neuropathy are absence of the normal sleep bradycardia and diminished variation of the pulse rate with inspiration-expiration or Valsalva (reduced sinus tachycardia), both due to early vagal involvement.

Later, sympathetic denervation interferes with normal cardiovascular reflexes, thereby diminishing exercise tolerance, possibly hypersensitizing the heart to circulating catecholamines, tachyarrhythmias, and sudden death. It also predisposes to painless myocardial infarction.

Orthostatic Hypotension

Accompanying orthostatic hypotension is managed by correcting hypovolemia with fluid replacement and improved diabetes control, elastic stockings, increased salt intake, mineralocorticoids, vasoconstrictors, a military antigravity suit, or atrial pacing.

Gastrointestinal Autonomic Neuropathy

Nonspecific gastrointestinal symptoms in diabetic patients often reflect diffuse but subtle gastrointestinal autonomic dysfunction. *Esophageal dysmotility* can cause dysphagia, retrosternal discomfort, and heartburn.

Delayed gastric emptying causes anorexia, nausea, vomiting, early satiety, and postprandial bloating and fullness. Delayed nutrient absorption can greatly complicate glycemic control, producing otherwise unexplained swings between severe hyperglycemia and hypoglycemia.

Diagnosis

Diagnosis of upper gastrointestinal symptoms requires liquid- and solid-phase radionuclide gastric-emptying studies. Diagnostic studies of lower gastrointestinal problems are necessary to define the multiple contributing factors that stem from widespread intestinal autonomic dysfunction to determine appropriate treatment.

Treatment
Management of esophageal dysmotility and delayed gastric emptying includes frequent small and/or primarily liquid feedings. High-fiber diets should be avoided, because they delay gastric emptying and may form bezoars. Dopamine antagonists such as metoclopramide or parasympathetic agonists may be helpful. A positive hydrogen breath test suggests bacterial overgrowth from stasis, and it supports a therapeutic trial of broad-spectrum antibiotics, whereas evidence of bile salt malabsorption would argue in favor of bile salt–sequestering agents, both of which are effective in properly selected patients. Hypermotility is managed with diphenoxylate hydrochloride.

Constipation
Diabetic constipation is the most frequent gastrointestinal complaint, occurring in 60% of patients with diabetes. Stool softeners and judiciously used laxatives or cathartics are usually effective, although dopamine antagonists are occasionally indicated. Diabetic diarrhea is classically painless, nocturnal, associated with fecal incontinence, and alternates with periods of constipation. Fecal incontinence, which is also usually nocturnal, reflects impaired sensation of rectal distention, and in one small series of patients it was effectively managed with biofeedback techniques.

Sexual Dysfunction

Erectile Impotence
Erectile impotence in diabetic men may be psychogenic, endocrine, vascular, drug, or stress related or neuropathic. (See **Coping,** Table 18, for questions to distinguish psychogenic impotence from other types.) Normal erections on awakening or impotence only with a certain partner suggests a psychogenic cause. A band-type turgidity gauge or nocturnal penile tumescence monitoring at a sleep research facility can help clarify ambiguous situations.

Sex steroid imbalances, hypogonadotrophism, and hyperprolactinemia should be excluded by appropriate endocrine studies. Proximal vascular insufficiency is usually evident on examination of the femoral pulses, although localized obstruction of the penile artery has been reported and can be excluded only by measurements of the brachial/penile blood pressure ratio using Doppler-flow studies. Proximal or localized vascular obstruction is surgically managed.

Drugs known to produce impotence include various antihypertensives, anticholinergics, antipsychotics, antidepressants, narcotics, barbiturates, alcohol, and amphetamines. Neuropathic impotence is generally but not always accompanied by other manifestations of diabetic neuropathy.

Management
Drug-induced impotence is managed by altering the treatment regimen when possible. Neuropathic impotence is managed by appropriate counseling and penile prostheses when indicated.

A nonsurgical technique involving a vacuum device and elastic constriction of the penis has been reported to be used successfully in men with diabetes, although its long-term safety is still being assessed. Injection of papaverine or other vasoactive drugs directly into the corpus cavernosum can stimulate erection in neuropathic impotence; however, this is an experimental approach.

Retrograde Ejaculation
Retrograde ejaculation, which may or may not occur in conjunction with impotence, reflects loss of the coordinated closure of the internal and relaxation of the external vesicle sphincter during ejaculation. Presentation is usually infertility, and diagnosis is confirmed by documenting ejaculate azoospermia and the presence of motile sperm in the postcoital urine. Such sperm have been successfully used for artificial insemination.

Other Autonomic Syndromes

Diabetic Cystopathy
Cystopathy initially diminishes sensation of bladder fullness, reducing urinary frequency. Later, efferent involvement produces incomplete urination, poor stream, dribbling, and overflow incontinence, and it predisposes to urinary tract infections.

Conservative management involves scheduled voluntary urination with or without Credé's maneuver, and cholinergic-stimulating drugs, sphincter relaxants, periodic catheterization, and bladder-neck resection of the internal sphincter may be used in more advanced cases.

Hypoglycemic Unawareness

Hypoglycemic unawareness is generally attributed to autonomic neuropathy of the adrenal medulla, which can blunt the usual adrenergic response to hypoglycemia. This is generally conceded to predispose to severe hypoglycemia and to be a major contraindication to intensive insulin treatment.

Autonomic Sudomotor Dysfunction

Autonomic sudomotor dysfunction produces an asymptomatic anhydrosis of the extremities and compensatory central hyperhydrosis. It diminishes thermoregulatory reserve and predisposes to heatstroke and hyperthermia. Management is confined to avoidance of heat stress.

FOCAL NEUROPATHIES

Neural deficits corresponding to the distribution of single or multiple peripheral nerves (mononeuropathy and mononeuropathy multiplex), cranial nerves, areas of the brachial or lumbosacral plexuses (plexopathy), or the nerve roots (radiculopathy) are relatively uncommon, of sudden onset, and generally but not always self-limiting in patients with diabetes.

Commonly, the third cranial nerve is affected, presenting with unilateral pain, diplopia, and ptosis but with pupillary sparing. Differential diagnosis includes an aneurysm of the internal carotid artery and myasthenia gravis. Spontaneous remission usually occurs within a few weeks.

Radiculopathy

Radiculopathy presents as bandlike thoracic or abdominal pain, often misdiagnosed as an acute intrathoracic or intra-abdominal emergency.

Femoral Neuropathy

Femoral neuropathy in patients with diabetes often involves motor and sensory deficits at the level of the sacral plexus as well as the femoral nerve, with the relative excess of motor versus sensory involvement differentiating diabetic femoral neuropathy from that seen in other conditions. When bilateral, this is sometimes termed *amyotrophy*. Management of focal neuropathies includes exclusion of other causes, e.g., nerve entrapment or compression and symptomatic palliation pending spontaneous resolution, which occurs generally but not always, over periods of months to years.

CONCLUSION

Diabetic neuropathy is an extremely common complication of diabetes that becomes more prevalent with increasing duration and severity of hyperglycemia. Its manifestations include diffuse and focal painful and painless neurological deficits in the peripheral nervous system and widespread autonomic dysfunction. Prompt and proper diagnosis is essential to effective management and avoidance of serious secondary musculoskeletal and visceral complications.

BIBLIOGRAPHY

Clements RS: Diabetic neuropathy: diagnosis and treatment. *Clin Diabetes* 2:73–92, 1984

Dyck PJ, Thomas PK, Asbury AK, Winegrad AI, Porte D (Eds.): *Diabetic Neuropathy*. Philadelphia, PA, Saunders, 1987

Greene DA, Lattimer SA, Sima AAF: Sorbitol phosphoinositides and Na-K ATPase in pathogenesis of diabetic complications. *N Engl J Med* 316: 599–606, 1987

Greene DA, Lattimer SA, Ulbrecht J, Carroll P: Glucose-induced alterations in nerve metabolism: current perspectives on the pathogenesis of diabetic neuropathy and future directions for research and therapy. *Diabetes Care* 8:290–99, 1985

Hilsted J, Richter E, Madsbad S: Metabolic and cardiovascular responses to epinephrine in diabetic autonomic neuropathy. *N Engl J Med* 317: 421–26, 1987

Macrovascular Disease

INTRODUCTION

Coronary heart disease, peripheral vascular disease, and cerebrovascular disease are more common and tend to occur at an earlier age and to be more extensive and severe in people with diabetes. Diabetes itself is a risk factor for atherosclerotic cardiovascular disease (ASCVD), most notably among women. Other risk factors include lipid abnormalities and hypertension, which are more prevalent in insulin-dependent (type I) diabetic individuals than in the general population, and cigarette smoking, which is as common among diabetic people as in the general population.

PREVALENCE AND RISK FACTORS

Although cardiovascular deaths are less common in type I diabetes than in the generally older patients with non-insulin-dependent (type II) diabetes, mortality rates among type I individuals are still more than 11 times greater than among individuals of the same age without diabetes. ASCVD accounts for approximately 25% of deaths among patients with onset of diabetes before 20 years of age. Heart disease causes 27% and strokes 6% of deaths among diabetic patients under 45 years old. A large percentage of these deaths result from the interaction of diabetes and hypertension, hypercholesterolemia, and cigarette smoking.

Diabetes is an independent risk factor for ASCVD, increasing risk two- to threefold. Diabetic women are at special risk. They do not seem to carry the normal "protection" of female gender, and their cardiovascular disease rates, even before menopause, parallel those of diabetic men.

Lipid abnormalities occur in 25 to 75% of adults, adolescents, and children with diabetes. Rates vary greatly depending on the characteristics of the study population, i.e., age, gender, type of diabetes, level of obesity, glycemic control, medications, and thyroid and renal status.

High levels of cholesterol and high ratios of total cholesterol to high-density lipoprotein cholesterol are powerful risk factors for cardiovascular disease; both are often elevated in type I patients, particularly in those with poor metabolic control. Triglyceride levels, another potential risk factor, are also generally higher in type I patients, especially during periods of hyperglycemia.

Hypertension and *cigarette smoking* are major cardiovascular risk factors. In health surveys of people 20 to 44 years of age, 29% of those with diabetes (compared to only 8% of those without diabetes) report having hypertension. In the same age groups, roughly 50% of people with diabetes report being cigarette smokers.

ASSESSMENT AND TREATMENT

Because of the high prevalence of risk factors, physicians should consider all patients with type I diabetes to be at risk for macrovascular disease. They should systematically assess patients for risk factors for ASCVD (those mentioned above plus a family history of cardiovascular disease or hyperlipidemia), question them about symptoms of ASCVD, and be alert for signs of atherosclerosis. When appropriate, a program for modifying risk factors should be started.

Hyperlipidemia

Hyperlipidemia in a diabetic patient may result from various causes, e.g., poor metabolic control, associated conditions such as hypothyroidism, or an independent inborn error of lipid metabolism. Each cause must be considered in assessing diabetic patients for high blood lipid levels.

The 1987 National Cholesterol Education Program (NCEP) guidelines recommend evaluation of fasting cholesterol levels in all adults over 20 years of age. For patients with diabetes, some physicians recommend screening cholesterol and triglycerides every 6 to 12 months in adults and prefer to begin screening in childhood. Fasting lipid levels should be assessed only when hypothyroidism has been excluded and the patient is in at least average blood glucose control.

If hyperlipidemia is present, the patient should be assessed for lipid-raising factors. Insulin treatment should be intensified because elevated triglyceride and cholesterol levels will return toward normal with intensification of insulin therapy in some minimally or poorly controlled patients. Any medications that might exacerbate hyperlipidemia, e.g., thiazide diuretics, should be discontinued, and the patient should be evaluated for renal disease and alcohol abuse. Genetic hyperlipidemias may be exacerbated by diabetes.

The physician should also determine whether the patient is following the current American Diabetes Association guidelines regarding fat intake (see **Nutrition,** Table 10).

Risk categories and recommendations for treatment can be found in Box 39. Implications for patients with diabetes are as follows.

- Men with total cholesterol over 200 mg/dl should be referred for lipoprotein analysis and treatment based on low-density lipoprotein cholesterol level (Box 40).
- Women with total cholesterol over 200 mg/dl *with* definite coronary heart disease or any risk factor or those with cholesterol over 240 mg/dl even *without* risk factors should be referred and treated as above.
- Women with total cholesterol over 200 mg/dl but without any risk factors or definite coronary heart disease should follow the dietary guidelines above and have cholesterol reexamined in 1 year.

Goals of therapy are to reduce serum cholesterol to 200 mg/dl or below and triglycerides to 150 mg/dl or below. Patients who exhibit persistent hyperlipidemia require more stringent dietary restriction and/or lipid-lowering drug therapy.

Box 39. Cholesterol Risk Categories and Recommendations for General Population

TOTAL CHOLESTEROL LEVEL (mg/dl)	RECOMMENDATION
<200 (desirable)	Repeat within 5 yr
200–239 (borderline high)	
Without definite coronary heart disease or 2 other risk factors*	Diet information, recheck annually; exclude hypothyroidism
With definite coronary heart disease or 2 other risk factors*	Refer for lipoprotein analysis; treat based on low-density lipoprotein cholesterol
≥240 (high)	Refer for lipoprotein analysis; treat based on low-density lipoprotein cholesterol

*Risk factors for coronary heart disease (CHD): diabetes; being male; high or borderline high blood pressure; family history of premature CHD; cigarette smoking; and severe obesity.

Adapted from the National Cholesterol Education Program: expert panel on detection, evaluation, and levels in adults. *Arch Intern Med* 148:36–69, 1988

Hypertension

Blood pressure should be measured in all patients with type I diabetes, including children and adolescents, at each physical examination—at least every 6 months—and hypertension treatment should be initiated to reduce the risk of microvascular and macrovascular disease. To the extent possible, blood pressure should be maintained at levels less than 140/90 mmHg in adults or below the 95th percentile for age- and sex-adjusted norms.

In prescribing therapy, the clinician should consider the adverse effects of various antihypertensive drugs on hyperglycemia and hypoglycemia, electrolyte balance, renal function, lipid metabolism, ASCVD, and neuropathic symptoms including orthostatic hypotension and impotence. (For a list of blood pressure–lowering medications, see **Nephropathy,** Table 19.)

Cigarette Smoking

Each patient's smoking history should also be determined. Nonsmokers, particularly children and adolescents, should be encouraged not to begin, and smokers should be strongly urged to stop. The physician's advice not to smoke has an impact and represents time well spent. Advice should be rein-

Box 40. Risk Categories Based on Low-Density Lipoprotein Cholesterol Levels

- Desirable: ≤130 mg/dl
- Borderline high risk: 130–159 mg/dl
- High risk: ≥160 mg/dl

Adapted from the National Cholesterol Education Program: Expert panel on detection, evaluation, and levels in adults. *Arch Intern Med* 148:36–69, 1988

forced with educational materials, referral to a smoking-cessation program, and by prohibiting smoking in the physician's office.

SYMPTOMS AND SIGNS OF ATHEROSCLEROSIS

The physician should be particularly alert to the symptoms and signs of atherosclerosis in all patients with diabetes.

Cerebrovascular Disease

Symptoms of cerebrovascular disease include intermittent dizziness, transient loss of vision, slurring of speech, and paresthesia or weakness of one arm or leg. Vascular bruits may be heard over the carotid arteries. Noninvasive procedures, including Doppler studies and CAT scans, may help to determine the diagnosis.

Aspirin at a dose of 325 mg daily may prevent a recurrence of symptoms, and use of anticoagulant medications for up to 3 months after a transient ischemic attack may help some patients. Angiography may be indicated when surgery is being considered, but the therapeutic value of surgical approaches to cerebrovascular disease has not been shown to be superior to standard medical therapy.

Coronary Heart Disease

As in people without type I diabetes, coronary heart disease may be associated with chest pain, shortness of breath, or congestive heart failure. However, among people with diabetes, ischemia may occur in the absence of chest pain (because of neuropathic damage to pain fibers to the heart). Unexplained onset of congestive heart failure and deterioration of glycemic control to the point of diabetic ketoacidosis may indicate silent myocardial ischemia, and myocardial infarction should be considered in the differential diagnosis of these conditions. Noninvasive procedures, including exercise tolerance tests, exercise thallium studies, and gated blood pool scans, may help establish the diagnosis of silent ischemia and/or myocardial perfusion defects.

Therapy may be medical or surgical. Medical treatments include aspirin, nitrates, calcium-channel blockers, and cardioselective beta-adrenergic blockers. Coronary angiography is necessary if bypass surgery or angioplasty is being considered. Bypass surgery or angioplasty is mandatory for left main coronary artery disease and is often indicated for triple-vessel disease, particularly in the presence of left ventricular dysfunction.

Peripheral Vascular Disease

Peripheral vascular disease should be suspected in patients who complain of buttock, calf, or thigh pain that occurs during exercise and is relieved with rest (intermittent claudication) and who exhibit decreased pulses in the lower extremities. The diagnosis can be confirmed with noninvasive Doppler studies.

Treatment with pentoxifylline may improve symptoms; aspirin and exercise are important adjuvants to treatment (see **Exercise,** p. 54 and Box 13). If pain is incapacitating or persists at rest or if a foot infection results from impaired blood flow through the major leg arteries, angioplasty or surgery to bypass the diseased vessels may be indicated. For more information on foot care see **Education,** p. 26, and **Neuropathy,** p. 126.

CONCLUSION

Patients with type I diabetes should be aware of their increased risk of ASCVD and advised of the importance of modifying risk factors such as hypertension, hyperlipidemia, and cigarette smoking.

Clinicians should systematically assess patients for risk factors for ASCVD and attempt to modify them. They should question patients about symptoms of ASCVD, examine them for signs of ASCVD, and seek the expertise of appropriate specialists when needed.

BIBLIOGRAPHY

Fielding JE: Smoking: health effects and control. *N Engl J Med* 313: 491–98, 555–60, 1985

Kannel WB, McGee DL: Diabetes and glucose tolerance as risk factors for cardiovascular disease: the Framingham study. *Diabetes Care* 2: 120–26, 1979

Lipid Research Clinics Program: The Lipid Research Clinics coronary primary prevention trial results. *JAMA* 251:351–74, 1984

National Cholesterol Education Program: Expert panel on detection, evaluation, and levels in adults. *Arch Intern Med* 148:36–69, 1988

Suarez L, Barrett-Connor E: Interaction between cigarette smoking and diabetes mellitus in the prediction of death attributed to cardiovascular disease. *Am J Epidemiol* 120:670–75, 1984

The Working Group of Hypertension in Diabetes: Statement on hypertension in diabetes mellitus: final report. *Arch Intern Med* 147:830–42, 1987

Limited Joint Mobility

INTRODUCTION

Limited joint mobility (LJM) is a potentially important *clinical marker for diabetes complications such as retinopathy, nephropathy, neuropathy,* statural growth abnormalities, hypertension, and hepatomegaly. Glycosylation of tissue proteins associated with chronic hyperglycemia may be responsible for many long-term complications, including LJM.

DETECTION AND EVALUATION

LJM may occur in children or adults, is painless, and causes minimal disability. Thus, it is unlikely to be brought to the attention of family members or health professionals. The only way to detect LJM is to examine hands and joints as part of routine office visits.

To evaluate for LJM the following should be included. Observe and shake both hands of the patient, noting any scleroderma-like stiffness of the skin. The patient should then be asked to place the hands in a clapping or "prayer" position with forearms as parallel to the floor as possible (Figure 15). Any inability to oppose the joints of the fingers and any limitation of flexion or extension of wrist, elbow, neck, or spine should be documented.

If pain or neuromuscular findings (e.g., atrophy, paresthesia) are present, other disorders such as tenosynovitis or carpal tunnel syndrome should be considered. In adults, another possibility is Dupuytren's contracture, which is painless and characterized by palmar nodules and involvement of the 3rd and 4th fingers.

Because there is a relationship between the severity of LJM and the microvascular complications of diabetes, patients found to have LJM at an office visit should be carefully examined for clinical evidence of retinopathy via ophthalmoscopy; for nephropathy by a quantitative determination of urinary protein excretion; and for hypertension, hepatomegaly, and neuropathy by careful clinical examination.

Figure 15. Limited Joint Mobility of Increasing Severity

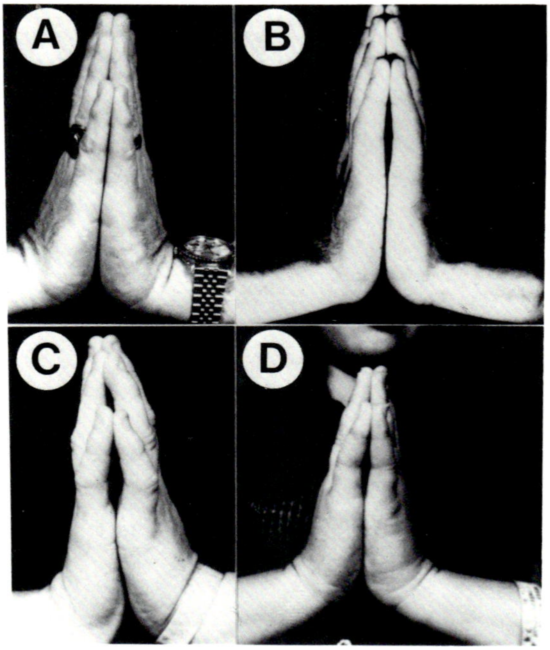

A: normal joint mobility. *B*: bilateral contracture of 5th fingers. *C*: bilateral contracture of more than 5th fingers. *D*: bilateral wrist involvement.

CONCLUSION

Until intervention in the primary glycosylation process becomes possible or better treatment strategies are perfected, patients with LJM should be periodically assessed for complications and should strive for the best possible glycemic control.

BIBLIOGRAPHY

Brink SJ: *Pediatric and Adolescent Diabetes Mellitus*. Chicago, IL, Year Book, 1987

Rosenbloom AL: Skeletal and joint manifestations of childhood diabetes. *Pediatr Clin N Am* 31:569–90, 1984

Growth

INTRODUCTION

Abnormalities of height (absolute short stature as well as decreased growth velocity) are known consequences of insulin deficiency. Although the classic example occurs in the extreme and relatively rare Mauriac syndrome (diabetic dwarfism), subtle abnormalities of growth and development are not uncommon among youngsters with insulin-dependent (type I) diabetes mellitus. The alterations usually result from inadequate metabolic control and can be prevented or corrected with better glycemic control.

MAURIAC SYNDROME

Children with Mauriac syndrome are markedly delayed in linear growth and sexual maturation. They are usually pale, appear chronically ill, and have a generalized puffiness of the face and extremities and a proturberant abdomen. Limited joint mobility and hepatomegaly are often present, and laboratory analysis includes not only hyperglycemia and elevated glycohemoglobin levels but also hyperlipidemia.

Figure 16. Inadequate Diabetes Control and Growth Abnormalities

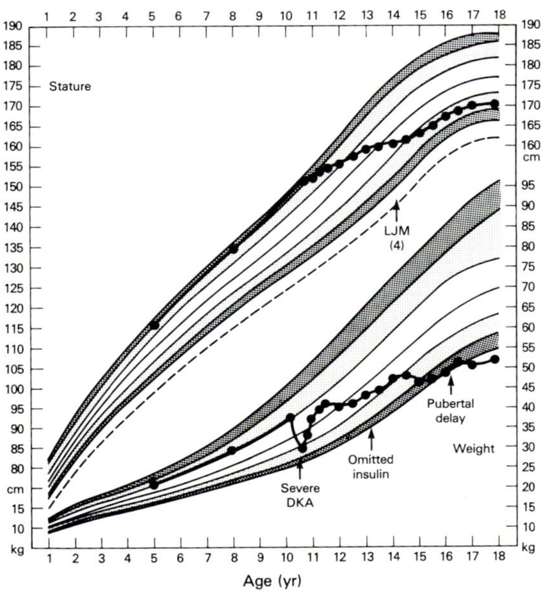

Growth deceleration solely from uncontrolled diabetes mellitus. Patient refused to take 2 shots of insulin each day. Most of the time, patient omitted morning insulin and refused to follow any type of meal plan. The family refused psychiatric consultation.

Adapted from Brink SJ: *Pediatric and Adolescent Diabetes Mellitus*. Chicago, IL, Year Book, 1987

SUBTLE GROWTH ABNORMALITIES

Less marked growth abnormalities become apparent when large patient populations are studied and subtle growth changes are sought, including a lag in height or weight or a deviation from previously established growth curves (Figures 16 and 17). Defined in this fashion, 5 to 10% of youngsters with type I diabetes will not grow well. Children most likely to be affected are those with the earliest onset of diabetes and those who have the worst day-to-day glycemic control and the highest glycohemoglobin levels. Boys are two or three times more likely to have a growth abnormality than girls.

DETERMINING GROWTH RATE

The only way to determine whether growth is adequate is to measure height and weight at each office visit and *to plot data on standardized growth charts.* Ideally, data should be recorded at least every 3 to 4 months but at least annually. Growth data obtained from other family members may be extremely valuable in placing an individual youngster's growth in perspective. Bone age determination (single radiograph of left wrist and hand compared with standard radiographs) coupled with other hormonal measurements may help assess the need for further evaluation. Other common diabetes-associated conditions should be considered as well (Table 21). If growth abnormalities are found, metabolic status should be carefully evaluated and appropriate recommendation for improvement made, such as changing from once- to twice-daily insulin injection.

Figure 17. Catch-Up Growth Phenomenon With Adequate Insulin

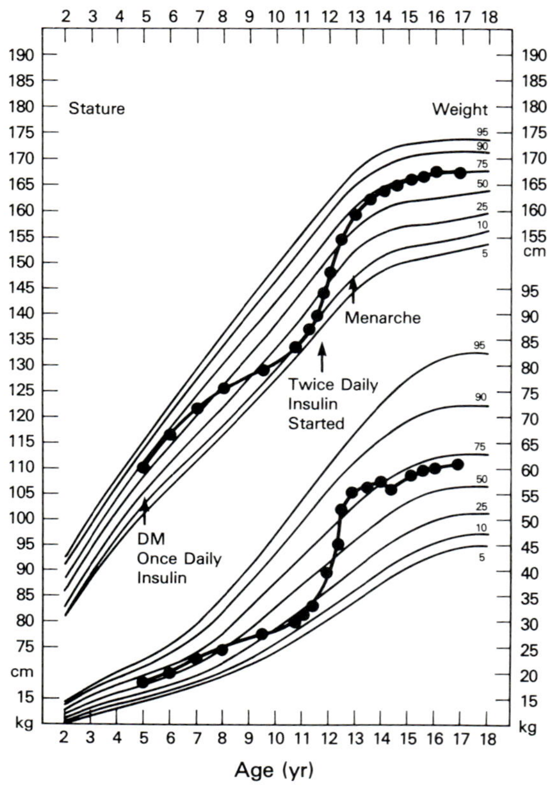

Growth data from child with type I diabetes treated with 1 shot of morning insulin, showing growth deceleration and catch-up growth phenomenon after twice-daily insulin was started.

Adapted from Brink SJ: *Pediatric and Adolescent Diabetes Mellitus.* Chicago, IL, Year Book, 1987

CONCLUSION

Although mild growth retardation may not be totally preventable, evidence strongly indicates that major alterations in growth rate can be avoided by better blood glucose control. Therefore, the definition of adequate diabetes control must include the attainment and maintenance of normal growth and development.

BIBLIOGRAPHY

Brink SJ: *Pediatric and Adolescent Diabetes Mellitus.* Chicago, IL, Year Book, 1987

Drash AL: Diabetes mellitus in the child and adolescent. II. *Curr Probl Pediatr* 16:500–501, 1986

Jackson RL, Guthrie RA: *The Physiological Management of Diabetes in Children.* New York, Medical Examination Publishing, 1986

Travis LB, Brouhard BJ, Schreiner BK: *Diabetes Mellitus in Children and Adolescents.* Philadelphia, PA, Saunders, 1987, p. 206–10

Affiliates

American Diabetes Association
ALABAMA AFFILIATE, INC.
3 Office Park Circle
Suite 115
Birmingham, AL 35223
(205) 870-5172; (205) 870-5173;
1-800-824-7891

American Diabetes Association
ALASKA AFFILIATE, INC.
201 E. 3rd Avenue
Suite 301
Anchorage, AK 99501
(907) 276-3607

American Diabetes Association
ARIZONA AFFILIATE, INC.
7337 North 19th Avenue
Room 404
Phoenix, AZ 85021
(602) 995-1515

American Diabetes Association
ARKANSAS AFFILIATE, INC.
Tanglewood Shopping Center
7509 Cantrell Road
Suite 227
Little Rock, AR 72207
(501) 666-6345

American Diabetes Association
CALIFORNIA AFFILIATE, INC.
2031 Howe Avenue
Suite 250
Sacramento, CA 95825
(916) 925-0199

American Diabetes Association
COLORADO AFFILIATE, INC.
2450 South Downing Street
Denver, CO 80210
(303) 778-7556

American Diabetes Association
CONNECTICUT AFFILIATE, INC.
P.O. Box 10160 (mailing address)
40 South Street
West Hartford, CT 06110
(203) 249-4232; (800) 842-6323

American Diabetes Association
DELAWARE AFFILIATE, INC.
2713 Lancaster Avenue
Wilmington, DE 19805
(302) 656-0030

American Diabetes Association
WASHINGTON, D.C., AREA AFFILIATE, INC.
1819 H Street, N.W.
Suite 1200
Washington, DC 20006
(202) 331-8303

American Diabetes Association
FLORIDA AFFILIATE, INC.
P.O. Box 19745 (mailing address)
Orlando, FL 32814
3101 Maguire Blvd., Suite 288
Orlando, FL 32803
(305) 894-6664

American Diabetes Association
GEORGIA AFFILIATE, INC.
3783 Presidential Parkway
Suite 102
Atlanta, GA 30340
(404) 454-8401

American Diabetes Association
HAWAII AFFILIATE, INC.
510 South Beretania Street
Honolulu, HI 96813
(808) 521-5677

American Diabetes Association
IDAHO AFFILIATE, INC.
1528 Vista
Boise, ID 83705
(208) 342-2774

American Diabetes Association
DOWNSTATE ILLINOIS AFFILIATE, INC.
965 North Water Street
Decatur, IL 62523
(217) 422-8228

American Diabetes Association
NORTHERN ILLINOIS AFFILIATE, INC.
6 North Michigan Avenue
Suite 1202
Chicago, IL 60602
(312) 346-1805

American Diabetes Association
INDIANA AFFILIATE, INC.
222 South Downey Avenue
Suite 320
Indianapolis, IN 46219
(317) 352-9226

American Diabetes Association
IOWA AFFILIATE, INC.
888 Tenth Street
Marion, IA 52302
(319) 373-0530

American Diabetes Association
KANSAS AFFILIATE, INC.
3210 East Douglas
Wichita, KS 67208
(316) 684-6091

American Diabetes Association
KENTUCKY AFFILIATE, INC.
745 W. Main Street
Suite 150
Louisville, Kentucky 40202
(502) 589-3837

American Diabetes Association
LOUISIANA AFFILIATE, INC.
9420 Lindale Avenue
Suite B
Baton Rouge, LA 70815
(504) 927-7732

American Diabetes Association
MAINE AFFILIATE, INC.
P.O. Box 2208 (mailing address)
c/o S. Parish Congregational Church
9 Church Street
Augusta, ME 04330
(207) 623-2232

American Diabetes Association
MARYLAND AFFILIATE, INC.
3701 Old Court Road
Suite 19
Baltimore, MD 21208
(301) 486-5516

American Diabetes Association
MASSACHUSETTS AFFILIATE, INC.
190 North Main Street
Natick, MA 01760
(617) 655-6900

American Diabetes Association
MICHIGAN AFFILIATE, INC.
The Clausen Building North Unit
23100 Providence Drive
Suite 475
Southfield, MI 48075
(313) 552-0480

American Diabetes Association
MINNESOTA AFFILIATE, INC.
3005 Ottawa Avenue, South
Minneapolis, MN 55416
(612) 920-6796

American Diabetes Association
MISSISSIPPI AFFILIATE, INC.
10 Lakeland Circle
Jackson, MS 39216
(601) 981-9511

American Diabetes Association
MISSOURI AFFILIATE, INC.
P.O. Box 1674 (mailing address)
213 Adams Street
Jefferson City, MO 65102
(314) 636-5552

American Diabetes Association
MONTANA AFFILIATE, INC.
P.O. Box 2411
Great Falls, MT 59403 (mailing address)
600 Central Plaza, Suite 304
Great Falls, MT 59401
(406) 761-0908

American Diabetes Association
NEBRASKA AFFILIATE, INC.
2730 South 114th Street
Omaha, NE 68144
(402) 333-5556

American Diabetes Association
NEVADA AFFILIATE, INC.
4550 East Charleston Boulevard
Las Vegas, NV 89104
(702) 459-7099

American Diabetes Association
NEW HAMPSHIRE AFFILIATE, INC.
P.O. Box 595 (mailing address)
Manchester, NH 03105
104 Middle Street
Manchester, NH 03101
(603) 627-9579

American Diabetes Association
NEW JERSEY AFFILIATE, INC.
P.O. Box 6423 (mailing address)
312 North Adamsville Road
Bridgewater, NJ 08807
(201) 725-7878

American Diabetes Association
NEW MEXICO AFFILIATE, INC.
525 San Pedro, N.E.
Suite 101
Albuquerque, NM 87108
(505) 266-5716

American Diabetes Association
NEW YORK DOWNSTATE AFFILIATE, INC.
505 8th Avenue
New York, NY 10018
(212) 947-9707

American Diabetes Association
NEW YORK UPSTATE AFFILIATE, INC.
P.O. Box 1037 (mailing address)
Syracuse, NY 13201
115 East Jefferson Street
Syracuse, NY 13202
(315) 472-9111

American Diabetes Association
NORTH CAROLINA AFFILIATE, INC.
2315-A Sunset Avenue
Rocky Mount, NC 27801
(919) 937-4121

American Diabetes Association
NORTH DAKOTA AFFILIATE, INC.
P.O. Box 234
Grand Forks, ND 58206-0234 (mailing address)
101 North 3rd St.
Suite 502
Grand Forks, ND 58201
(701) 746-4427

American Diabetes Association
OHIO AFFILIATE, INC.
705L Lakeview Plaza Court
Columbus, OH 43085
(614) 436-1917

American Diabetes Association
OKLAHOMA AFFILIATE, INC.
Warren Professional Building
6465 South Yale Avenue
Suite 423
Tulsa, OK 74136
(918) 492-3839 or 1 (800) 722-5448

American Diabetes Association
OREGON AFFILIATE, INC.
3607 S.W. Corbett Street
Portland, OR 97201
(503) 228-0849

American Diabetes Association
GREATER PHILADELPHIA AFFILIATE, INC.
21 South Fifth Street
The Bourse
Suite 570
Philadelphia, PA 19106
(215) 627-7718

American Diabetes Association
MID-PENNSYLVANIA AFFILIATE, INC.
2045 Westgate Drive
Suite B-1
Bethlehem, PA 18017
(215) 867-6660

American Diabetes Association
WESTERN PENNSYLVANIA AFFILIATE, INC.
4617 Winthrop Street
Pittsburgh, PA 15213
(412) 682-3392

American Diabetes Association
RHODE ISLAND AFFILIATE, INC.
4 Fallon Avenue
Providence, RI 02908
(401) 331-0099

American Diabetes Association
SOUTH CAROLINA AFFILIATE, INC.
P.O. Box 50782 (mailing address)
2838 Devine Street
Columbia, SC 29250
(803) 799-4246

American Diabetes Association
SOUTH DAKOTA AFFILIATE, INC.
P.O. Box 659 (mailing address)
Sioux Falls, SD 57101
1524 West 20th Street
Sioux Falls, SD 57105
(605) 335-7670

American Diabetes Association
TENNESSEE AFFILIATE, INC.
1701 21st Avenue, South
Room 403
Nashville, TN 37212
(615) 298-9919

American Diabetes Association
TEXAS AFFILIATE, INC.
8140 North Mopac
Building 1
Suite 130
Austin, TX 78759
(512) 343-6981

American Diabetes Association
UTAH AFFILIATE, INC.
643 East 400 South
Salt Lake City, UT 84102
(801) 363-3024

American Diabetes Association
VERMONT AFFILIATE, INC.
217 Church Street
Burlington, VT 05401
(802) 862-3882

American Diabetes Association
VIRGINIA AFFILIATE, INC.
404 8th Street, N.E.
Suite C
Charlottesville, VA 22901
(804) 293-4953

American Diabetes Association
WASHINGTON AFFILIATE, INC.
3201 Fremont Avenue North
Seattle, WA 98103
(206) 632-4576; 1-800-628-8808

American Diabetes Association
WEST VIRGINIA AFFILIATE, INC.
Professional Building
1036 Quarrier Street
Room 404
Charleston, WV 25301
(304) 346-6418; 1-800-642-3055

American Diabetes Association
WISCONSIN AFFILIATE, INC.
10721 W. Capitol Drive
Milwaukee, WI 53222
(414) 464-9395

American Diabetes Association
WYOMING AFFILIATE, INC.
2908 Kelly Drive
Cheyenne, WY 82001
(307) 638-3578; (307) 237-2325

Index

A

B

C

D

E

F

G

H

N

P

R

S

T

V

Publications of the American Diabetes Association

PROFESSIONAL PERIODICALS

Diabetes

The leading U.S. basic research journal on diabetes, presenting the latest laboratory findings from the world's most eminent scientists. Published monthly. Price $70.00 for 1 year US/Canada; $105 for 1 year International.

Diabetes Care

Now published 10 times a year. *Diabetes Care* offers clinicians and researchers the latest research findings that relate to diagnosis, diet, exercise, monitoring, drug therapy, and complications and their management. Price $55.00 for 1 year US/Canada; $82 for 1 year International.

Clinical Diabetes

ADA's bimonthly newsletter of current clinical information and practical applications to patient care. Easy-to-read format. Price $15.00 for 1 year.

IDF Bulletin

International news on diabetes research and treatment. Published for the International Diabetes Federation. Price $20.00 for 1 year; 3 issues per year.

NEW

Diabetes Spectrum

This new bimonthly publication focuses on the latest research advances and translates them into "what this means to your practice." *Diabetes Spectrum* is designed for every member of the diabetes health-care team. Price $30.00 for 1 year US/Canada; $40 for 1 year International.

PATIENT PERIODICALS

Diabetes Forecast

A colorful monthly magazine that focuses on living with diabetes from the patient's perspective. *Diabetes Forecast* provides the latest information to help patients better understand and control diabetes. Price $20.00 for 1 year US/Canada; $33.00 for 1 year International for 12 issues plus membership in the ADA.

FREE

Diabetes '88/'89

A free quarterly newsletter that addresses important questions patients have on diet, exercise, self-monitoring, research advances, and life-style. Free bulk quantities can be ordered for distribution to patients. Indicate how many you need per quarter on the order form in back. Available in the US only.

CLINICAL EDUCATION PROGRAM (CEP)

REVISED AND UPDATED

Physician's Guide to Non-Insulin-Dependent (Type II) Diabetes: Diagnosis and Treatment—Second Edition

This newly revised handbook, designed for primary-care physicians and other health-care professionals, is updated to answer the complex questions encountered in treating non-insulin-dependent diabetes mellitus. It is the one practical reference manual you need to resolve problems. Covers diagnosis, pathogenesis, management, and complications. 112 pages. Spiral-bound. 1988
#037 Nonmember: 22.45;
Member: $18.45

Forty Commonly Asked Questions About Type II Diabetes (NIDDM)
This booklet was developed from hundreds of questions collected from attendees of the CEP and answered by CEP's expert panel. It provides you with a handy and practical instructional tool. 36 pages. Softcover. 1984 #036 Nonmember: $3.75; Member: $3.00

NEW

Clinical Diabetes Reviews, Volume I
This new book covers the most important topics in the treatment of diabetes, including diagnosis, pathogenesis, drug therapy, routine management, and special problems and complications. It is especially designed for the physician and health-care professional who spend less than 50% of his/her time with diabetic patients. *CDR* is a compilation of articles (1983–1987) from *Clinical Diabetes* and *Diabetes Care*. 200 pages. Softcover. 1987 #408 Nonmember: $19.95; Member: $15.95

Goals for Diabetes Education
This book covers all the goals and objectives of effective diabetes education in an easy-to-use checklist format. 48 pages. Softcover. 1987 #201 Nonmember: $6.00; Member: $4.80

OTHER PROFESSIONAL PUBLICATIONS

Curriculum for Youth Education
A guide for diabetes educators that outlines patient education goals for youth, detailing objectives and expectations for each age group. *While supplies last*. 88 pages. Softcover. 1983 #505 Nonmember: $7.00; Member: $5.60

Third-Party Reimbursement for Diabetes Outpatient Education: A Manual for Health-Care Professionals
This useful publication was developed by the ADA Task Force on Financing Quality Health Care. If your organization is seeking reimbursement for an outpatient education program, this paper is a must. 18 pages. 1986 #225 Nonmember: $2.00; Member: $1.60

Diabetes Outpatient Education: The Evidence of Cost Savings
This paper stresses the importance of patient education as an effective treatment program and provides rationale for third-party reimbursement. 6 pages. 1986 #226 Nonmember: $.50; Member: $.40

ORDER TODAY!

To place your order, make your check or money order payable in U.S. dollars, drawn on a U.S. bank, to the American Diabetes Association, Attn: Order Dept., 1660 Duke St., Alexandria, VA 22314. Be sure to include the item no., title, quantity, price, and total for each publication. If you are an ADA member and would like to take advantage of the Member's Price, make sure you indicate your membership number (appears on your *Diabetes Forecast* label) on the order. All prices include shipping and handling charges and are subject to change without notice. Allow 6 to 8 weeks for domestic delivery and add appropriate time for foreign surface delivery.

American Diabetes Association, Inc.

Publisher
CAROLINE STEVENS

Director of Professional Publications
BEVERLY BRITTAN COOK

Managing Editor
ORIT LOWY CHICHERIO

Medical Writer
DOROTHY SEGAL

Project Editor
ARLENE KARIDIS

Design Coordinator
STEPHEN J. CHICHERIO